THE EAT FAT, GET THIN
COOKBOOK

THE EAT FAT, GET THIN COOKBOOK

More Than 175 Delicious Recipes for Sustained Weight Loss and Vibrant Health

Dr Mark Hyman

Food photography by Leela Cyd

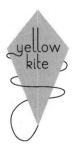

yellow kite

First published the USA in 2016 by Little, Brown and Company
Hachette Book Group Inc

First published in Great Britain in 2016 by Yellow Kite Books
An imprint of Hodder & Stoughton
An Hachette UK company

1

Trade Paperback ISBN 978 1 473 65380 1
Ebook ISBN 978 1 473 65381 8

Food stylist: Ayda Robana
Food photographer: Leela Cyd

Printed and bound by Clays Ltd, St Ives plc

Hodder & Stoughton policy is to use papers that are natural, renewable and recyclable products and made from wood grown in sustainable forests. The logging and manufacturing processes are expected to conform to the environmental regulations of the country of origin.

Hodder & Stoughton Ltd
Carmelite House
50 Victoria Embankment
London EC4Y 0DZ

www.hodder.co.uk

This book is dedicated to anyone who has suffered through a low-fat diet. It's time to eat food that tastes good and is good for you.

Contents

Contents

THE EAT FAT, GET THIN
COOKBOOK

Introduction

I've seen thousands of patients just like Joanne—people who have tried countless diets and exercise plans, yet have been unable to achieve their health goals. That's because typical diets don't work.

I know that might sound crazy, but hear me out. Typical diets combine calorie deprivation with tasteless foods, which is a recipe for failure. It's simply too hard to keep cravings at bay when you feel deprived and aren't enjoying the food you do eat. Sugar addiction always seems to rear its ugly head, causing people to fall off the wagon. The problem with most diets is that they lack the key ingredient that actually makes food taste good and cuts your hunger: fat!

This is what makes the *Eat Fat, Get Thin* Plan different from other diets. It's not about deprivation or bland foods; it's about eating foods that nourish the whole body, while making your taste buds happy and fixing the hormones that make you hungry and gain weight.

Decades of brainwashing have left many of us afraid of one of the body's most necessary nutrients. I can't tell you how many patients I've had to coach, using baby steps, to eat coconut oil and avocados, or how many people have come to my house and been horrified to see me blending grass-fed butter into my coffee. I understand these responses, since I, too, had fat phobia at one point. I spent years eating a low-fat diet and recommending it to all my patients. The idea of promoting fat, especially saturated fat, in a healthy diet seemed outrageous.

It's not hard to understand where this fat fear came from. For years, doctors, scientists, the media, and even our government told us that eating fat causes weight gain and heart disease. These two myths, based on a few faulty studies, started a huge war on fat. Fats were soon replaced by carbs, sugar, and chemicals ("low fat" is usually code for "high sugar"), leading to one of the worst disease epidemics of all time. Type 2 diabetes in the UK has doubled since 1996, and researchers estimate that five million Britons will have diabetes by 2025.

We now know that sugars and carbs, not fats, are the true causes of obesity and heart disease. Overconsumption of processed carbohydrates causes a spike in the body's production of the hormone insulin, which increases the storage of fat, especially dangerous belly fat. And that is just the start of the damage that sugar can do to your body.

Dietary fat, on the other hand, does not cause a spike in insulin. Unlike eating carbs, eating fat makes your body burn fat, rather than store it. Fats like butter and coconut oil, which were once maligned, are now being touted for their metabolism-boosting properties and the way they suppress hunger, lower triglycerides, reduce fat storage, and even improve athletic performance. Olive oil, or what I like to call liquid gold, has been shown to prevent heart disease, cancer, and diabetes. Healthy fats—such as avocados, wild fatty fish, nuts and seeds, and coconut and olive oils—also reduce inflammation in the body, help your brain perform better, and increase your overall energy. When you make healthy fats part of a low-glycemic (low sugar and starch), real- and whole-food diet, you can absolutely heal your body.

Digging through the research on fat over the last ten years has been life-changing for me, in my practice and in my personal life. When I started to recommend fat to my own patients, I saw some of them lose one hundred or more pounds and even reverse type 2 diabetes. I had never witnessed such dramatic transformations before.

I began including more fats in my diet as well, and I noticed a shift in my own health. After getting off processed carbs and increasing my fat intake, not only did I have more mental focus and clarity, but I lost fifteen pounds and my love handles turned into a six-pack without my exercising any more than I had previously. I'm now eating more calories and losing more weight, and I eat fat with every single meal! For breakfast I'll often have an omelet or a frittata cooked in grass-fed butter, or a smoothie made with nuts and seeds, coconut milk, and/or an avocado. For lunch I might have a big salad with wild fatty fish like salmon or sardines, plus avocados and pumpkin seeds with plenty of extra-virgin olive oil, and for dinner, grass-fed lamb (keeping the fat on it, of course) paired with different veggies and more olive oil on top. The satisfaction of eating increases dramatically when you cook your food with real, healthy fats. Fat is what makes food taste good.

With the help of my friend Chef Frank Giglio, I've put together more than 175 deeply satisfying and delicious recipes to share with you. You can use these recipes before, during, and after your twenty-one-day *Eat Fat, Get Thin* Plan, which you can find in my book *Eat Fat, Get Thin* and in Part II of this book. I've also included recipes that are specifically designed to be used after the twenty-one-day plan. They fall into what I like to call the Pegan Diet. The Pegan Diet, which I explain in Chapter 4, combines the best of the Paleo and vegan diets. It is the way that I eat 90 percent of the time, and I've never felt better. I'm sharing the recipes in this book because I want everyone to feel this way—satisfied, satiated, and full of energy and vitality.

Let's take back our kitchens and take back our health. It all starts in these pages.

PART I

THE BASICS

So many of you have already experienced monumental changes in your health. Some of you may just be getting started, and others might be looking for a reset to get back on track. Wherever you are on this journey, I hope this cookbook serves as inspiration to continue to seek the best version of yourself. In these next chapters, I'll give you my best tips for creating a safe and joyful space for healing and thriving, and we'll recap the *Eat Fat, Get Thin* Plan, so that you feel fully prepared to enthusiastically and easily take control of your health.

1

Seven Big Ideas

Before we get started with the *Eat Fat, Get Thin* Plan, I want to take you through some key principles that have helped me and my patients on the journey to optimal health. You might be familiar with some of these concepts, and in that case, consider them helpful reminders. Some are related to food, others are more about emotional health, but all are necessary on the path toward vibrant well-being. I call them the Seven Big Ideas.

BIG IDEA 1: FOOD IS NOT LIKE MEDICINE — IT *IS* MEDICINE

Nothing beats the true healing power of real food. Normally, by the time patients come to a Functional Medicine doctor like me, they've exhausted what conventional medicine offers. Conventional medicine is by far the best for acute illness. But food is the best medicine for chronic disease. It works faster and better, and is cheaper than medication. And all the side effects are good ones. Remember Joanne's story—off insulin, diabetes medication, and blood-pressure medication in four days after fifteen years of struggling. No drug can do what (real) food can do.

Nutrigenomics is the idea that food is information and that that information is always communicating with our genes, turning on messages that foster health and/or disease. If every part of each food we eat contains valuable information for our bodies that affects gene expression, then why, for so long, were we obsessed with focusing only on one tiny part of the food we consume: the number of calories? Calories matter, but far less than the information or instructions in food that control our

9

genes, hormones, immune system, enzymes, and even our gut flora or microbiome with every single bite.

Imagine what message you're sending your body when you eat nutritionally empty foods such as cheeseburgers, potato chips, French fries, and cupcakes. Compare this to the message sent by plant foods, which are packed with powerful antioxidants and phytochemicals that your body needs. Unfortunately, there are some foods, like fat, that continue to be demonized even though they send important and very powerful messages to our cells.

A decade ago, when I started to really dig into the research on dietary fats, I found undeniably clear evidence that in the absence of refined sugars and processed carbohydrates, healthy fats shut down cravings, speed up metabolism, and can help prevent and reverse heart disease, *not* cause it. But because we were (and still are) a country focused on calories, and because fats contain more calories than processed carbohydrates or sugars, many "experts" continued to dismiss this macronutrient because it is more "calorie dense." I'm happy to report that several recent studies have shown how incredibly powerful and healing good fats are and that saturated fat is *not* the villain it was made out to be for so long. And that fat actually helps you lose weight, not gain weight. We need to put dangerous low-fat diets behind us as we embrace the fact that we have the most healing treatments in the world available right at our fingertips, and they come from the "farmacy," not the pharmacy.

BIG IDEA 2: FOOD AND FAT ARE *NOT* THE ENEMY

Our relationship with food is one of the most important relationships in our lives. It's also one of our first relationships. From day one, food nourishes us and enables us to live and thrive. But like any long-term relationship, this one can become toxic. Sadly, fear around food and fat is more prevalent than ever. We have been convinced that fat makes us fat and that all calories are equal and should be counted as such. But metabolism is not a math problem. It is about the quality and composition of our food and the hormones and molecules they influence.

Before you start the twenty-one-day plan, I want you to take out your journal or a piece of paper and really think about your relationship with food and fat. Ask yourself the following questions:

- What beliefs am I holding on to about fat?
- What is my relationship to or belief about a fat-free diet?
- How have low-fat diets worked for me in the past? What happened when I tried them?
- What worries or fears do I have about including fat in my diet?

Answering these questions is the first step in letting go of any negative relationship with food and fat. If you are a chronic dieter, the *Eat Fat, Get Thin* Plan is perfect for you. Once you clear out the junk and reset your body, you can move on to a way of eating that allows room for pleasure foods while focusing on eating real, whole foods most of the time. You'll be able to think of food as a friend who nourishes you and brings you joy instead of an enemy you have to fear or battle every day.

BIG IDEA 3: BE YOUR OWN DOCTOR

Conventional medicine focuses on naming diseases based on specific body location instead of underlying cause. Doctors say you have liver, kidney, brain, or heart disease, but this approach tells you nothing about the *cause*.

Instead of asking what disease you have and what drug should be used to treat it, we must ask what underlying causes led to the disease or illness. I empower my patients to do a little bit of investigative work specific to them, because no two bodies are the same. One person's weight gain might be the result of mercury toxicity, while another's stems from imbalances in gut flora that have led to irritable bowel syndrome. Become a detective.

What works for your neighbor might not work for you. Some people do better with a higher-fat diet and others do better with more carbs such as sweet potatoes or small amounts of whole grains (no one does well on lots of processed carbs or flours). Experiment with these foods, and while you experiment, keep track of your findings in a food journal, taking note of how you feel after your meals. Your body will give you clues each day. Inquisitiveness and intuition will help you discover where your ailments are coming from and what might help treat them. We just have to listen and pay attention.

BIG IDEA 4: WEIGHT LOSS — EVERYONE IS DIFFERENT

Eat Fat, Get Thin is more than a catchy title—it's the truth. Dietary fat can actually speed up your metabolism and help you lose weight. Even better, once you start this program, you'll find that it's a gateway to something much bigger than the numbers on the scale.

Weight loss happens differently for everyone. You might find that you lose more weight in the beginning of the program or at the end, or it might happen steadily all the way through. We're all different and have different paces and needs. Be patient with your body. Make sure you're drinking enough water and moving your bowels every day. Get at least thirty minutes of exercise a day (ideally including high-intensity interval training) to speed up your metabolism and to get the endorphins flowing; they lift your mood and make challenges seem less daunting. Endorphins make you feel good, and when you feel good, you tend to make healthier choices for your body. Also, recognize that weight loss might take some time. Three weeks can create a huge shift in your body, but it's still just three weeks. Depending on how many years of poor eating, lack of exercise, or other issues have preceded the program, we may have to dig deeper. Environmental toxins, nutritional imbalances, hormonal imbalances, a damaged gut, and stress can all contribute to unexplained weight gain. A program like *Eat Fat, Get Thin* is a great starting point, but if you suspect that there is a deeper issue, or if you're struggling along the way, I recommend seeking the help of a Functional Medicine practitioner (Royal London Hospital for Integrated Medicine, www.uclh.nhs.uk/ourservices/serviceA-Z).

BIG IDEA 5: ASK WHY

Learn more, love more, be a better doctor, be a better father, reach more people, heal the planet, end obesity. These are just some of my personal goals, and my desire to achieve these goals is what motivates me to put my health first. Anytime I feel stressed and fail to adequately take care of myself, I always stop and remember why. Why is my health important? My health is important because I can't show up as the best version of myself and go after my goals if I feel sick, unhealthy, unbalanced, or stressed.

Before you start this program, and as you go through it, I want you to ask yourself *why* you're doing it. Maybe you want to increase your energy so that you can keep up with your kids or grandkids, or perhaps you want more mental clarity to perform better at work or school. Maybe you want to feel good in your own skin so you can have better relationships with the people you love. Whatever they are, it's essential to remind yourself of your own personal goals on a daily basis. Not only are they more achievable when you feel energized, but you get to enjoy the journey as you work toward them, which is just as, if not more, important.

The first step is really clearly setting your goals. Ask yourself what's important to you and how you can live in ways that are in alignment with this vision. I have never met anyone who wakes up in the morning and says, "It's my goal to get fatter and sicker and create disease." So, odds are this is not your goal; therefore, why would you make choices that lead to this outcome? Chances are, you want the complete opposite for yourself. You want to feel good, look good, and cook delicious and healthy meals that make you feel satisfied. You want to prepare this food and share these benefits with the people in your life as well, so how can you make decisions that support this outcome? You want to design your life to create health and well-being, not disease or "feeling like crap." Think about how you can redesign your life to make healthy choices automatic.

Just sticking with the recommendations of this plan is not always enough to keep the motivation going, but taking a look at your goals and reminding yourself of the bigger picture will help you to keep your perspective.

BIG IDEA 6: FRIEND-POWER, NOT WILLPOWER

In 2014, I wrote *The Daniel Plan* with my friends Pastor Rick Warren and Dr. Daniel Amen. We took Pastor Warren's congregations through a six-week challenge based on the principles of Functional Medicine to change biology and optimize health and the power of social connections and positive peer pressure to change behavior. We used the power of social networks to hold people accountable and help them reach their health goals.

The results were astounding. The congregations lost 115,000 kilos in ten months. They also improved things like depression, autoimmune disease, diabetes, high blood pressure, and acne. One day, Pastor Warren said, "Every *body* needs a buddy. Getting healthy is a team sport." Those words stuck with me. The reason we experienced such profound results during our first trial of The Daniel Plan was because the congregation was playing as a team.

Instead of using willpower, I recommend using friend-power. If you can do this program with a family member or friend, that's awesome! You can also start a community meet-up for intentional eaters in your area, find a coach, or join our online community (www.drhyman.com /community). You may be surprised at how many people have been wanting to change their habits but were waiting for someone else to encourage them. Creating a community of like-minded people will always lead to a more favorable outcome for everybody, as group encouragement goes a long way. Humans are pack animals and social creatures; we're meant to rely on one another for support.

Granted, you may occasionally run into a naysayer who feels threatened by the lifestyle changes you're making. I call these "food pushers." Just have that one piece of cake—*what's the big deal?* they say. I find that people who react negatively to my eating habits often behave that way because they are questioning their own diet and lifestyle. It can be hard, but try to take the high road. Stick to what feels good, trust that you are making the best decisions for yourself, and don't pay any attention to what the haters say. In fact, as you're making changes, now might be a good time to (gently) cut the negative energy loose.

BIG IDEA 7: LEAVE THE JUDGMENT BEHIND

I recently came across this quote: "If you had a friend who talked to you the way that you talked to yourself, you would have ditched that friend a long time ago." How true is that? We are our own harshest critics. So I challenge you to now become your own best friend. Instead of looking in the mirror and judging yourself for everything you believe to be wrong with your body, why not praise yourself for taking this huge step toward better health?

Your body is listening to everything you say. Indulging in self-deprecation leads to stress; stress wreaks havoc on your health. And if you find yourself making a bad decision or going off course during this journey, leave the guilt behind, too. It's just as toxic, and it doesn't help you at all. Be like your car's GPS: when you veer off course, gently remind yourself to make a U-turn. The diet and exercise industry is filled with borderline harmful messages like "no pain, no gain," and we have been taught that looking good has to feel bad. Killing ourselves at the gym, forcing ourselves to eat foods we find unenjoyable, or, even worse, starving and denying ourselves is a recipe for disaster.

I encourage you, instead, to find joy in this process. Joy makes food taste better. Every single recipe in this book has been created and taste tested for maximum pleasure and flavor. I am not an advocate of suffering to become the best version of yourself. The best version of yourself is healthy *and* happy. The best version of yourself loves to be active, play in the sunshine, and create beautiful, wholesome meals. This collection of recipes is designed to nourish that best version of you, with recipes that make your mouth water *and* make you feel good.

Everyone's path is different, but we are all in this together. If you are reading this book, you are interested in bettering yourself, and that's incredibly exciting. Know that the road to your own personal vibrant health can absolutely be enjoyable.

Now that we've prepared our minds, it is time to prepare our kitchens!

Be sure to talk with your health care provider before embarking on this journey, especially if you're on any medications or dealing with chronic illness.

2

Getting Started: The *Eat Fat, Get Thin* Plan

In the recent documentary series *Cooked*, my friend Michael Pollan discussed the correlation between time spent in the kitchen and obesity rates. No surprise here: As the average amount of time that we spend in the kitchen has gone down, obesity rates have gone up. I understand where the desire to outsource cooking comes from; my schedule is pretty jam-packed, and some days even the thought of walking into the kitchen can be daunting. But what is the cost of choosing convenience over real nourishment? A sick nation. A world in which families are disconnected and spending more time in front of their TVs or hunched over a screen, mindlessly eating processed takeout, and less time with one another eating real food. And the truth is that simple cooking doesn't take a long time, and it is not inconvenient or expensive. It is a bunch of propaganda the food industry has convinced us is true. Anyway, how convenient or cheap is it to be sick and fat and tired and have chronic diseases and take medication your entire life? Not so much!

The only way to ensure that you and your family are eating safe, nutritious food is to get back into the kitchen and make the time to connect with what you're eating. You should be able to identify every single ingredient in your meals and snacks. Think about how long it took for that ingredient to get from the farm to your fork. If it made a pit stop at a factory, or if it was made in a factory, and sometimes even if it sat on a truck for days traveling across the country to get to you, it may not be good enough for your body. Remember, you deserve real food. It's a birthright of being human.

The first step to reconnecting with your kitchen is to make it a safe zone by filling it with foods that nourish and removing foods that harm. This will ensure that you automatically make the right choices, especially if you're pressed for time and looking for something quick. The same goes for your backpack, purse, car, school locker, and so on; anywhere you look for food, you should have only the good stuff available. Think of all the willpower it takes to have to battle cravings for junk food that's right under your nose, and all the other places that energy could go instead! Set yourself up for success by making your home and environment a safe zone free of foods that harm you and make you feel bad, and full of foods that heal and make you feel good.

The first part of the *Eat Fat, Get Thin* Plan is the preparation stage, which I recommend starting two days before your program. This involves giving your kitchen a makeover so that you can prepare these flavorful meals quickly and easily and complete your twenty-one-day *Eat Fat, Get Thin* Plan with success. Even if you're using this book just for recipes, I still recommend detoxifying your kitchen, as it makes it so much easier to choose healthy options.

Next, I'll cover everything that you'll eat and drink during the twenty-one-day plan, and finally, I'll lay out the Pegan Diet, which is the diet that you'll transition to after the twenty-one-day plan.

Thousands of people have participated in the *Eat Fat, Get Thin* Plan, and they've experienced significant weight loss, a decrease in cravings, and balanced blood sugar and blood pressure, as well as a *huge* reduction in symptoms of many different diseases and health issues. That is how powerful this program is, and it all starts with the food that we eat. The benefits come from using food as medicine to create health. The pounds and symptoms drop off as side effects.

So let's get started with your kitchen makeover. Have your trash bag and recycling bin ready to completely remove all of the following items from your cupboards and fridge:

- Anything containing hydrogenated oils or refined vegetable oils (like corn or soybean). These oils are highly unstable and inflammatory. We were told that vegetable oils were healthy alternatives to butter and lard, but they actually contribute to heart disease, diabetes, cancer, and a number of other ailments. Get rid of them. Bonus: Getting rid of these ingredients means you pretty much eliminate all packaged and processed foods, since most of them contain these oils. So you're eliminating excess sugar and salt in one fell swoop! The average salad dressing is made from soybean oil and high-fructose corn syrup. What a way to ruin your vegetables!

- All fake foods. Get rid of anything that's processed or contains preservatives, additives, or dyes. Get rid of anything labeled "fat free" or "low fat" or "natural flavors," which are not really natural at all. Those words almost always mean that sugar or additives have taken the place of healthy fat.

- Anything containing artificial sweeteners (Splenda, sorbitol, aspartame, etc.) or processed sugar, especially high-fructose corn syrup.

- All processed meats, such as deli meats. The World Health Organization has singled these out as major causes of disease, including cancer.

While the above items are toxic and should be avoided completely, you might be able to incorporate some of the following foods back into your diet after the twenty-one-day plan. But you'll want to keep them out of sight for three weeks:

- Any product containing gluten. An undiagnosed gluten intolerance can cause a whole host of problems, including autoimmune conditions, leaky gut, dementia, and diabetes. Most of us generally feel better when we avoid it, especially in the highly processed and often chemical- and GMO-filled gluten products in this country. And the main form we consume gluten in is flour, which is worse than table sugar and is highly addictive.

- Non-gluten grains. These include rice, quinoa, barley, millet, or any other grains. Whole grains can be a wonderful part of a healthy diet, but they are still starch and can spike blood sugar and insulin. They also create gut problems and inflammation for some people, so we avoid them during the first twenty-one days of the program.
- All dairy products. Dairy is often full of hormones and antibiotics. The only dairy I recommend is grass-fed butter or ghee, and some people do okay with raw cheese, yogurt, or milk from pastured animals, but save those personal experiments until after the twenty-one days. Ideally, use ghee — which removes the casein and whey (the allergenic proteins in dairy).
- Beans. They contain a fair amount of starch, and for blood sugar issues, they aren't ideal. They can also cause digestive problems, something we're trying to avoid on the program.
- All fruit, with the exception of berries, pomegranate seeds, watermelon, lemons, limes, and kiwi. Fruit is full of antioxidants, beneficial fiber, and nutrients, but I have seen plenty of patients overindulge in fruits as a substitute for their sugary snacks. When you're trying to lose weight or balance your blood sugar, it's best to stick with a small amount of low-glycemic fruit. A good rule of thumb is to eat primarily fruit that's local and in season, which drastically limits the amount of fruit we eat for most of the year. Remember, the natural packaging that fruit comes in has a purpose, as nature always knows what it's doing! When you do eat fruit, try to eat the pith and the skin, too, as the added fiber slows down blood sugar and the bitterness of the pith aids in digestion.
- All alcohol. Regular alcohol consumption can cause inflammation, which can lead to weight gain, pre-diabetes, and diabetes. It also creates strong and often uncontrollable cravings and can put a large strain on your gut and liver health. Use in moderation (three to five drinks per week at most) once you're done with the program, but avoid alcohol for these three weeks.

FILL YOUR FRIDGES AND STOCK YOUR PANTRIES

Now that you've removed the poison from your pantries (or the foods that can sabotage your health), we can talk about all of the delicious foods you'll get to eat every day. When creating a healthy meal or snack, there are three types of foods to focus on. It's more about all the good, delicious things you can eat rather than the things you can't.

- First: slow carbs or nonstarchy plant foods. These include green leafy veggies, broccoli, mushrooms, tomatoes, peppers, bok choy, and many, many more. When it comes to slow carbs, the options are endless. These foods should make up 75 percent of your plate. I place an emphasis on nonstarchy veggies because they contain potent antioxidants, vitamins, and minerals that have powerful healing properties and are low in sugar or starch. On the *Eat Fat, Get Thin* Plan you can occasionally include starchy veggies (beetroot, parsnips, sweet potatoes, and yams) for dinner.
- Second: protein. On average, you should be getting 100 to 175 g of protein with each meal. This is about the size of the palm of your hand. Protein is necessary for appetite control and muscle synthesis. Muscle is your metabolic engine. Your protein sources will come from free-range eggs, nuts and seeds, grass-fed and organic meats, clean fish, and non-GMO whole soy foods.
- Last but certainly not least: fats. The right fats can improve your mood, skin, hair, and nails, while protecting you against type 2 diabetes, dementia, cancer, and much more. Healthy fats are the best source of energy for your body and keep your metabolism and fat-burning mechanism running as they're meant to. And they are the key to cutting cravings and curbing your appetite. Be sure to eat at least four to five servings of fat per day. Healthy fats can be found in foods like wild fatty fish (sardines, mackerel, herring, wild salmon), grass-fed meat or organic poultry (skin and fat left on), nuts and seeds, avocados, extra-virgin olive oil, and coconut oil.

Here are some examples of a fat serving:

- Extra-virgin coconut oil (1 tablespoon)
- Extra-virgin olive oil, avocado oil, macadamia oil, walnut oil, almond oil (1 tablespoon)
- MCT oil (page 27, 1 to 2 tablespoons a day)
- Organic coconut milk (60 ml)
- Avocado (½ to 1 avocado)
- Fatty fish like sardines, mackerel, herring, black cod, and wild salmon (100 to 175 g); aim to include these three to four times per week
- Nuts and seeds (2 to 3 handfuls)
- Olives (60 ml cup)
- Grass-fed butter, clarified butter, or ghee (1 tablespoon); if you are allergic to dairy, just use ghee

The following is a cheat sheet listing all the approved foods and fats and the off-limits ones. You can photocopy these pages and keep them in your purse or wallet, or take a picture with your smartphone, and use them for easy reference when you're at the shops.

Going Organic

When possible, choose organic, seasonal, and local produce. To help you prioritize when choices are limited, consult the Environmental Working Group's "Dirty Dozen" and "Clean Fifteen" lists, showing the foods you should always source organic due to pesticide use and/or skin thickness, and those you can safely buy when organic isn't an option. The expanded "Dirty Dozen" list includes apples, celery, sweet peppers, peaches, strawberries, nectarines, grapes, spinach, lettuce, cucumbers, blueberries, potatoes, grapes, kale, and all other green leafy veggies. Don't forget about the freezer section; you can often find organic fruits and vegetables there. Check out www.ewg.org for an updated list.

What to Eat		
	Focus on These Items…	Avoid These Items…
Fat (aim for 4 to 5 servings a day, all organic)	Nuts (except for peanuts), seeds, and nut butters: chia, flax, sesame, black sesame, sunflower, hemp seeds, pumpkin seeds, hazelnuts, macadamia nuts, pecans, walnuts, almonds, cashews Nut and seed milks: almond, Brazil nut, cashew, coconut, hemp Avocados, olives Ghee, grass-fed butter, coconut butter Oils (extra-virgin and cold-pressed): avocado, coconut, macadamia nut, MCT (page 27), olive, walnut, sesame	Dairy products (except for grass-fed butter and ghee; those are okay) (for 21 days) All refined vegetable oils: corn, rapeseed, safflower, soy, sunflower (for the long term)
Animal foods/ protein (aim for 100 to 175 g of protein per meal, all grass-fed and organic). Can also be vegetable protein in the form of non-GMO whole soy.	Bison, beef, elk, lamb, ostrich, venison Eggs, chicken, duck, turkey Lard, tallow, duck and goose fat (free-range, pasture-raised) Fresh or canned fatty fish: black cod, herring, mackerel, perch, sardines, scallops, wild salmon, anchovies Shellfish: clams, crab, mussels, oysters, prawns, scallops Non-GMO tofu, tempeh	Legumes, beans (for 21 days) Processed meats: bacon, canned meats, hot dogs, salami (for the long term) High-mercury fish: king mackerel, tuna, swordfish, Chilean sea bass, halibut, lobster, marlin, shark, tilefish, orange roughy (for the long term). See www.nrdc.org for a guide to low-mercury fish.
Carbohydrates (raw, steamed, roasted, or sautéed; approximately 50 to 75 percent of your plate should be made up of nonstarchy veggies)	Artichokes, asparagus, aubergines, avocados, bean sprouts (not alfalfa sprouts, which contain natural carcinogens), beetroot greens, broccoli, Brussels sprouts, cabbage, carrots (no juicing because it turns them into pure sugar), cauliflower, celery, chard, chives, courgettes, dandelion greens, endive, fennel, fresh herbs, garlic, ginger, green beans, hearts of palm, jalapeño cillies, kale, lettuce, mangetout,	Gluten, all grains (for 21 days) All fruit (with the exception of berries, kiwi, lemon, lime, pomegranate seeds, watermelon: 75 to 150 g per day) (for 21 days)

	Focus on These Items…	*Avoid These Items…*
Carbohydrates *(continued)*	mushrooms, mustard greens, onions, radicchio, radishes, rocket seaweeds (kelp, arame, wakame, etc.), shallots, sugar snap peas, spinach, spring greens, summer squash, sweet peppers, tomatoes, turnip greens, watercress 100 to 150 g of starchy veggies up to 4 times a week at dinner: beetroot, celeriac, parsnips, pumpkin, sweet potatoes, winter squash (butternut, kabocha, acorn, etc.)	
Drinks	Hot lemon water, sparkling water with lemon or lime, herbal or green teas, Bulletproof Coffee or Tea, bone broth	Alcohol (for 21 days) Fizzy drinks (including 'diet' types), milk, fruit juices, sports drinks (for the long term)
Other (condiments, spices, staples)	Almond flour, apple cider vinegar, arrowroot, balsamic vinegar, black peppercorns, coconut flour, coconut aminos, Dijon mustard, kelp noodles, kimchi, miso, nutritional yeast, organic vegetable and chicken stock, sea salt, spirulina, tahini, ume plum vinegar, unsweetened vanilla and chocolate (cacao) powder, wheat-free tamari, dried or fresh herbs and spices such as basil, cayenne pepper, chili powder, cinnamon, coriander, cardamom, ginger, cumin, onion powder, oregano, paprika, parsley, rosemary, sage, thyme, turmeric	Natural sweeteners: honey, maple syrup, raw sugar, etc. (for 21 days) Additives, preservatives, dyes, MSG (for the long term) Artificial sweeteners: Splenda, Equal, acesulfame-K, aspartame, mannitol, saccharin, sorbitol, xylitol, stevia (for the long term)

Some of the items listed in the approved section might be unfamiliar, but I promise that experimenting with them is well worth it. For example, we've included a recipe for pancakes (page 82) that uses coconut flour instead of regular flour. Trust me, you don't want to miss out on these pancakes! New and different ingredients help spice up your cooking routine so you're not stuck with the same few meals day after day. Let me introduce you to some of the new ingredients you will experiment with.

Almond Flour and Almond Meal

An alternative to grain-based flours, almond flour is made by blanching and grinding almonds into a fine powder. Almond meal is typically a coarser grind made with the skin still left on. Both can be used to bake breads, desserts, and pastry cases. They are full of protein and good fats, as well as vitamins and minerals.

Apple Cider Vinegar

I use apple cider vinegar in my salad dressings, sauces, and dips. It is anti-bacterial and antiviral, it helps combat constipation, and it can make your skin glow when taken daily.

Arrowroot

Arrowroot is a thickener that can be used in soups, stews, baked goods, and more. It is a great alternative to conventional thickeners like cornflour.

Bone Broth

Bone broth contains powerful gut-healing properties. Chicken, beef, lamb, bison, venison, turkey, and/or duck bones are simmered for long periods of time with veggies and filtered water to create an immunity-supporting beverage that can be sipped on its own or added to other meals, soups, and stews. Great for kids, pets, and anyone with compromised digestion. You can get the recipe on page 128.

Bulletproof Coffee

Coffee is not a requirement on this program, but if you do enjoy coffee, Bulletproof Coffee, invented by my friend Dave Asprey, will change your life with its frothy goodness. Adding fat to your coffee can stop cravings and improve brain function and focus. To Bulletproof your beverage, blend 250 ml coffee, 1 tablespoon of grass-fed butter or ghee, 1 tablespoon of coconut or MCT oil, and, if you like, ½ teaspoon of cinnamon and/or cocoa powder (for a mocha). If you aren't a coffee fan, you can also add fat to your tea using the same recipe. If you want to be dairy free, you can use 1 table-spoon of organic cashew butter, which makes it creamy and delicious.

Chia Seeds

These tiny black seeds pack an antioxidant punch and are filled with omega-3 fatty acids and fiber to help feed friendly gut bacteria. They can be added to smoothies and, since they absorb water easily, also used to create puddings. We have a yummy recipe for chia seed pudding on page 87.

Coconut Aminos

Coconut aminos are a terrific alternative to soy sauce. They are made from coconut sap and have a similar consistency and taste to soy sauce, but they are gluten-free. They also contain minerals as well as vitamins B and C and can be used in stir-fries, soups, dips, and more. You can find them in your local health-food store or online.

Coconut Butter

Coconut butter is made from the meat of coconuts, and it has a thick, buttery consistency that I love using in my smoothies as a thickener. I also spread it on homemade, grain-free breads for a super-satiating snack. You can find it in the nut-butter section of most grocery stores or online.

Coconut Cream

An amazing whipped cream alternative! Coconut cream has a higher fat con-tent than coconut milk, so you can whip it into a rich texture to top ice creams or add to your coffee drinks. A Bulletproof Coffee with whipped coconut cream is the most amazing (and healthy) treat! Go for an organic brand, such as Native Forest, Biona or Tiana, which you can purchase online or at health-food stores.

Coconut Flour

Just like almond flour, coconut flour makes a great substitute for grain-based flours. It is made from dried coconut flesh, and is a bit sweeter than almond flour, so it's great for sweet breads and pancakes. It's an excellent source of fiber and helps balance blood sugar and eliminate cravings.

Flaxseed

Also know as linseed, flax seed is an ideal source of essential omega-3 fats, dietary fiber, and key vitamins and minerals. I like adding it to my smoothies and salads. It also helps to combat constipation and keep blood sugar levels in check. Keep refrigerated, especially if the seeds are ground.

Ghee

Also known as clarified butter, ghee is made by melting butter, then simmering it over low heat until most of the water evaporates and the milk solids float to the top to be skimmed off, leaving beneficial fat. In Ayurvedic medicine, ghee is used for its powerful healing properties. It's perfect for high-temperature cooking since it stays stable at high heats. You can find a recipe for ghee on page 279.

Grass-fed Butter

The only other dairy product I recommend is grass-fed butter. Beef from cows that are fed only grain produces a much higher omega-6 content in comparison to grass-fed cows, and since omega-6 fats are more inflammatory, I suggest sticking to grass-fed butter. It's great for satiation, energy, and improved mood and brain function.

Hemp Seeds

Hemp seeds are gaining in popularity and with good reason, as they are a true powerhouse of nutritional benefit. They are a fantastic source of protein, iron, and magnesium. You can sprinkle them onto your salads or add them to your smoothies and baked goods.

Kelp Noodles

Ditch the pasta for good! Kelp noodles are a nutritionally dense alternative to grains, made from kelp, a kind of seaweed. They're really mineral-rich, so you can enjoy them without guilt. We've included a couple of kelp noodle recipes for you to try out.

Kimchi

Fermented foods have been rising in popularity over the years as gut health has taken center stage. Kimchi is a traditional Korean food that involves fermenting a variety of vegetables with probiotics. The result is a fiber- and nutrient-rich dish that can be cooked with other ingredients or served raw as a side (for the most gut benefit).

MCT Oil

MCT stands for medium-chain triglycerides, a fatty acid derived from coconut oil. Consider MCT oil a superfuel for your cells because it boosts fat burning and increases mental clarity. You can use it in your coffee and add it to smoothies, salads, or any other meal. You can find MCT oil on our resources page at www.eatfatgetthin.com/resources.

Miso

Fermenting soybeans creates this immunity-boosting superfood that can be used to make soups, sauces, and dressings. There are many different kinds of miso. Look for the ones that are fermented without grains.

Nutritional Yeast

Believe it or not, cheesy, creamy salads and sauces can be achieved without using dairy. Nutritional yeast is deactivated yeast that you can sprinkle onto your meals. It's one of my favorite condiments because it adds a delicious flavor and a cheesy texture, and it's a great source of energy-providing vitamin B_{12}.

Spirulina

A blue-green algae that's a wonderful source of B vitamins, protein, and iron, spirulina is another powerhouse food that can be eaten by meat eaters and vegetarians alike. Listing all of the benefits of spirulina would take up a whole page—let's just say I highly recommend it. I personally love to add it to smoothies and on top of salads, and a tiny bit goes a long way.

Tahini

Made from ground sesame seeds, and high in protein and healthy fat, tahini (alone or blended with other ingredients) makes the perfect dressing or dip for your vegetables. It's a great alternative to nut butters, especially for those who are allergic to nuts.

Teff Flour

Teff flour is a gluten-free flour made from a grain called teff and is traditionally used in Ethiopian cuisine to make bread. Teff is rich in protein, calcium, and iron. We've included a delicious bread made from teff in the recipes (page 253). You can find teff flour in health-food stores and online.

Tempeh

Made from fermented soybeans, tempeh has a dense texture with a good amount of protein, so if you're vegetarian or looking to experiment with a new food, try replacing the animal protein in recipes with tempeh. Fermented tempeh is a healthier alternative to processed soy products like tofu and TVP (textured vegetable protein).

Ume Plum Vinegar

Ume plum vinegar is made from fermented umeboshi plums. It has a unique salty-sour taste and can be used as a general seasoning or in soups, stocks, sauces, and stir-fries. It's also traditionally used as a detoxification aid and palate cleanser.

Wheat- and Gluten-Free Tamari

Instead of using soy sauce, try wheat-free tamari. It has a similar taste and is a significantly healthier, gluten-free option.

STOCK YOUR TOOLBOX

Experimenting with all of these delicious foods is much easier and a lot more fun when you have the right tools. Think of these tools as an investment in your health. Once I equipped myself with a great set of knives, a powerful blender, wooden cutting boards, and other quality kitchen essentials, I was much more excited about playing in the kitchen. The following tools are essential:

Blender (if you can afford it, I recommend getting a VitaMix; it will last a lifetime)

Good set of knives (keep them sharp)

2 wooden cutting boards (one for animal foods, one for fruits and vegetables, and some people like to keep a third for onions and garlic)

Nonstick sauté pan, cast-iron pan, or both

8-litre stockpot

2-litre and 4-litre saucepans with lids

Several rimmed baking sheets

Several square and/or rectangular baking dishes

Food processor (sometimes a blender can be used instead, but a food processor is a handy kitchen tool to have as well)

Instant-read thermometer

Spatulas (metal and rubber)

Can opener

Colander

Measuring jugs, metal for dry ingredients and glass for liquids

Measuring spoons

Mixing bowls

Wooden spoons

The following tools make cooking a little easier, but they are optional. You definitely don't have to go out and spend a ton of money and overhaul your kitchen to make this program work for you.

30-cm square nonstick pan griddle
Flameproof casserole dish (suitable for oven and hob)
Grill pan
Steamer
Coffee grinder for flaxseeds and spices
Vegetable-steaming rack or basket
Citrus reamer (for extracting juice by hand)
Rubber spatulas
Balloon whisks
Spring tongs
Pliers or tweezers (for deboning fish)
Microplane graters/zesters in assorted sizes
Food mill
Natural baking parchment and foil
Tea towels
Spiralizer (for making vegetable noodles)
Mandolin slicer
Vegetable peeler
Timer (most everyone's phone has one now)
Sealable glass containers in various sizes for storing food (preferred to plastic storage containers, as they don't leach plastic into your food)

STOCK YOUR MEDICINE CABINETS

Eating real, whole foods, and especially plant foods, is the most important part of your transformation toward optimal health. In the long run, plant foods are the best source of vitamins, minerals, phytonutrients, antioxidants, and fiber, but because of depleted soils, the vegetables and fruits we eat have fewer nutrients than plants grown in healthy organic soils.

Foundational support through supplementation is key to healing your gut, reducing inflammation, balancing blood sugar, and recovering from nutritional deficiencies. Here's a rundown of all the supplements you will need for your twenty-one-day plan (and they can be taken over the long term as well to maintain your health). You can purchase these as a full pack for ease and convenience at www.eatfatgetthin.com/resources, or purchase them individually at your local health-food store.

Supplement	Benefits	Daily Dosage
High-quality multivitamin and multimineral	*Contains all the B vitamins, antioxidants, and minerals you need to help run your metabolism and improve blood sugar and insulin functioning*	Follow the manufacturer's label instructions for dosage. Most good multivitamins and minerals require 2 to 4 capsules or tablets a day to obtain adequate doses.
Purified fish oil (EPA/DHA)	*Acts as an anti-inflammatory, insulin- and blood sugar-balancing, heart disease-preventing, brain-boosting supplement*	2 to 4 grams a day
Vitamin D_3	*Helps insulin function*	2,000 to 4,000 units a day
L-carnitine	*Assists with fat-burning for fuel*	300 to 400 milligrams twice a day
Coenzyme Q10 (antioxidant)	*Helps to optimize energy production and supports heart health*	30 milligrams twice a day
PGX fiber (superfiber)	*Slows blood sugar and insulin spikes and can also cut cravings and promote weight loss*	2.5 to 5 grams just before every meal with a large glass of filtered water. Can be taken as powder or softgels.
Magnesium glycinate (relaxation mineral)	*Helps to reduce anxiety, improve sleep, assist blood sugar control, cure muscle cramps, and help with constipation*	100 to 150 milligrams (2 to 3 capsules once or twice a day)

(continued)

Supplement	Benefits	Daily Dosage
Probiotics	*Helps normalize your gut flora*	10 to 20 billion CFU (colony-forming units)
MCT oil (superfat from coconut oil)	*Speeds up your metabolism, improves liver function, and fuels your brain*	1 to 2 tablespoons a day
Electrolytes (E-lyte) (combination of electrolytes and salt); optional	*Helps with proper tissue hydration and makes you feel amazing*	1 to 2 capfuls a day
Potato starch; optional (I recommend Bob's Red Mill Unmodified Potato Starch, available at most local health-food stores)	*A form of "resistant starch" that helps balance your blood sugar and feed the good gut bugs, both of which help with weight loss*	Build up to 1 to 2 tablespoons in 250 ml of filtered water twice a day

A TYPICAL DAY ON *EAT FAT, GET THIN*

Now that you've stocked your kitchen with nutritious foods and the right tools and supplements, you're ready to start the twenty-one-day plan. The full plan can be found in my book *Eat Fat, Get Thin*, but here's a snapshot:

Morning

- Begin the day with 30 minutes of movement (walking or other exercise)
- Before breakfast, take 2.5 to 5 grams of the PGX fiber (1 to 2 packets or ½ to 1 scoop of the powder in 300 ml of filtered water, or 3 to 6 capsules)
- Take your supplements with breakfast
- Take your MCT oil or add it to your coffee or smoothie
- Make and eat your smoothie or breakfast
- Optional: Have a midmorning snack (you can find snack recipes beginning on page 88)

- Drink water (at least 8 glasses throughout the day); use at least 1 capful of E-lyte in 250 ml of filtered water twice a day to help with proper hydration

Afternoon

- Before lunch, take 2.5 to 5 grams of the PGX fiber
- Eat lunch
- Optional: Have a midafternoon snack
- Drink water (at least 8 glasses throughout the day)

Evening

- Before dinner, take 2.5 to 5 grams of the PGX fiber
- Eat dinner
- Optional: Have 1 tablespoon of potato starch in water before bed
- Get 7 to 8 hours of quality sleep

It's as easy as that. But I promise, three simple weeks can drastically change your life.

3

Tips, Tips, and More Tips

I've put together a few tips that will enhance your three-week experience and beyond, on everything from grocery shopping to cooking with fats to preparing meals for the kids. I use these tricks to get the most out of my food and my time, and they have made me feel less stressed about putting healthy meals on the table every day.

TIP 1: HOW TO MAKE THE MOST OF YOUR FATS

I want to touch briefly on cooking with fats since they are the main focus of this plan. Fat is complicated. Unlike sugar, different fats interact with your body in different ways. For example, trans fats increase inflammation, while omega-3 fats reduce inflammation. Some fats destabilize when heated, so they become toxic to the body when cooked, while other fats remain stable at higher temperatures and can actually enhance the vitamin and mineral assimilation in different ingredients. Here are a few easy tips that will maximize the amount of nutrition you get out of your food.

Oils

Knowing which oils to use, and what to use them for, is the key to experiencing their benefits.

Coconut oil, sesame oil, avocado oil, and ghee are best for higher-heat cooking, as they have a higher smoke point and do not become toxic as quickly as other oils when exposed to heat. Olive oil is best for low-heat cooking or, used raw, for dressing salads. Macadamia oil and walnut oil also are wonderful raw and make great dressings.

With all oils, always choose organic, unrefined, cold-pressed, or expeller-pressed (which involves some heat) . Be sure to do your research, and don't be afraid to contact the company directly to ensure that the product is truly cold-pressed. Organic production prohibits GMOs and the use of hexanes for extraction in oils.

Store oils in dark, not clear, bottles and keep in a cool, dark place away from light and heat. Don't store oils on kitchen counters or next to the stove because they will oxidize or turn rancid. Always close the lid tightly, and immediately store oils after using them because oxygen contributes to rancidity. Oils go bad over a span of months depending on type. That's why it is so important to purchase only the amount you will use within two months. Choose good-quality organic brands of oil, such as Biona, Tiana and Clearspring, and be sure to check out the most competitive prices online.

Animal Fats

Grass-fed and pasture-raised animals live in cleaner, healthier, and more sustainable environments compared with intensively reared animals. That's why I always recommend buying grass-fed *and* grass-finished beef (meaning the animal has been raised on grass for its entire life) whenever possible.

The meat and dairy from intensively reared animals have less nutritional benefit for us and contain harmful additives and contaminants such as antibiotics, hormones, and pesticides. The animals are fed diets of genetically modified (GMO) grains, corn, barley, and soybeans to speed up weight gain. Studies have linked the consumption of genetically modified food (including meat) to serious health risks in humans, such as infertility, immunity problems, faster aging, improper insulin function, and changes in vital organs, including the gastrointestinal system. Intensively reared animals are often given antibiotics and growth hormones, so when we eat their meat, we are also exposed to these.

When animals suffer, the whole planet suffers. It's an undisputed fact that healthy and happy animals make for healthy meat. I like to get my meats from local farms so I can talk to the farmers about the way the animals were raised and see their living conditions and food with my own eyes if possible. It is important to choose your meats wisely to receive their full nourishing benefits and take responsibility for the lives of the animals that provide the food we consume.

Fish and Seafood

Fish and seafood are the absolute best sources of complete omega-3 fatty acids, EPA and DHA, but toxic mercury levels make it vital to choose fish from the best possible source. I personally suffered from mercury toxicity as a result of growing up on tuna fish sandwiches, eating a ton of sushi, and having a mouth full of amalgam fillings. I felt tired and weak all the time. I suffered from depression, anxiety, digestive problems, and other debilitating symptoms. Mercury toxicity is one of the most prevalent ailments that I see in my practice. Avoiding fish high in this heavy metal is of the utmost importance.

According to the Environmental Working Group, the best sources of omega-3 fish that also contain the lowest levels of mercury are wild salmon, sardines, mussels, rainbow trout, herring, anchovies, and Atlantic mackerel. The fish we should avoid are king mackerel, lobster, marlin, tuna, halibut, Chilean sea bass, orange roughy, shark, swordfish, and tilefish. To avoid toxic exposure, we should choose wild and high-quality fish sources whenever possible.

Nuts and Seeds

Everyone who knows me knows that I am nuts for nuts and seeds! They make the perfect snack or topping for your salads, and they are filled with healthy fats and vitamins and minerals that can improve your hormones, your brain health, and your heart health. However, nuts and seeds also contain phytates, which bind to important minerals, such as iron, zinc, magnesium, and calcium, and limit absorption of these minerals from the digestive tract. These minerals play a critical role in preventing diabetes and obesity, and a deficiency in them is often seen with type 2 diabetes.

Soaking and rinsing raw nuts and seeds effectively reduces the phytates and enzyme inhibitors.

Soaking is a pretty simple process: soak raw nuts or seeds in warm salt water (1 tablespoon of salt for 400g of nuts or seeds) overnight or for up to twenty-four hours. Make sure the nuts and seeds are fully submerged in the water. Once they are finished soaking, rinse them off thoroughly. It's important to let them dry fully so they don't mold. Lay them out in the sun or spread them on a pan and place in the oven on a warm setting, no more than 50°C/120°F (if necessary, leave the door ajar to get this low temperature and use an oven thermometer to monitor it). With a dehydrator, you can set the heat setting to no more than 42°C/108°F and still preserve most nutrients. Dehydrate or leave in oven for twelve to twenty-four hours.

TIP 2: HOW TO EAT WELL ON A BUDGET

When I was a junior doctor, I had to support a wife and two kids on $27,000 a year. I have met families all over the world with limited finances, and they were still able to eat well on a budget. It is absolutely possible with a little bit of planning, and you're still going to be able to enjoy delicious and flavorful meals, I promise. Here are my eating-for-less strategies:

1. Ditch the processed and packaged foods! Good news: you will already be doing this on the *Eat Fat, Get Thin* Plan. In terms of price per nutrient density, fruits and veggies are way less expensive than packaged foods. I also recommend avoiding "healthy" packaged foods. These are the boxes and bags that line the shelves at your health-food store. They are usually overpriced and often full of sugar, even if it is organic cane sugar. Plus, if you take a look at the ingredients, you'll find you can quite often just as easily make these foods at home. Kale chips require a few spices, some oil, and an oven. While you're at it, skip the coffee queues, too. Even buying just one coffee a day adds up fast, and combining all those convenience-food purchases, you might be shocked at how much

you're spending and how easy it is to make healthier alternatives in your own kitchen. Write down how much money you spend on little things every day, expenses you could avoid and that would save you money for real food.

2. Hit the discount stores. Aldi and Lidl stock organic products, often far cheaper than at other grocery stores. Also try various online stores and compare prices. Among those offering good value are Healthy Supplies (www.healthysupplies.co.uk) and Real Foods (www.realfoods.co.uk).

3. Learn to love and prepare at least five to ten basic recipes. Keep ingredients for these recipes around at all times so that you can quickly make them when you're in a bind or low on time. You can also save money by freezing meats and leftovers so they don't go bad.

4. Buy in bulk and stock up when you see a sale on your favorite storable foods. Don't forget, you can freeze a lot of foods or ingredients that you won't use right away. People who live in rural areas often find that a chest freezer is a wise investment if trips to the grocery store are infrequent.

5. Check out the NHS guide to budget food shopping (www.nhs.uk/livewell/eat4cheap) and the BBC budget menu (www.bbcgoodfood.com/feature/budget).

TIP 3: HOW TO GROCERY SHOP WITH EASE

Shopping for healthy and delicious foods can be done just about anywhere. You don't have to have access to farmers' markets, gourmet-food stores, or even health-food stores. You can go to your regular grocery store and usually find what you need, and it doesn't take very long either. Also, don't be afraid to ask your local grocery store to stock specific items for you. The more people ask, the more likely the store is to bring new items in, and even if you're the only person asking for it, you might be pleasantly surprised at how accommodating the store is. So if you don't see organic almond butter or organic produce, ask for it!

The first step is to make a shopping list. This obviously saves you from wandering the aisles aimlessly and subsequently purchasing junk food on impulse. The second step is to stick to the outside aisles, or, more specifically, the produce section, for your main ingredients, and remember, when selecting beef or meat, choose grass-fed, hormone-free, or organic, when possible. Next, load up on the following essentials, which will make cooking (and healthy choices) easier:

- Extra-virgin olive oil
- Extra-virgin coconut oil
- Other favorite oils, such as walnut, sesame, flax, and avocado
- Nuts, such as walnuts, almonds, pecans, and macadamias
- Seeds, such as hemp, chia, flax or linseed, pumpkin, and sesame
- Unsweetened nut milk
- Almond flour and coconut flour
- Canned full-fat coconut milk, unsweetened
- Kalamata olives
- Apple cider vinegar
- Balsamic vinegar
- Bone broth (homemade or low-sodium chicken or vegetable stock)
- Dijon mustard
- Sea salt
- Freshly ground black pepper
- Seasonings and spices, such as cayenne, cinnamon, chili powder, cumin, curry powder, garlic powder, oregano, onion powder, paprika, parsley, rosemary, sage, thyme, and turmeric
- Wheat-free tamari (low-sodium)

Most of these staples can be found at big discount stores, but some might not be available at your grocery store, or they may be unreasonably priced. That's when online shopping can be very useful. Try the websites for Healthy Supplies and Real Food.

TIP 4: HOW TO SAVE TIME

When you're short on time, it is incredible how a little bit of strategic planning goes a very long way.

Frozen fruits and vegetables are key time-savers. I like to stock my freezer with frozen berries, vegetables, grass-fed beef, and wild salmon.

I also recommend buying prewashed and precut veggies (organic, of course) if you're short on time. This will help you cut down on time spent prepping in the kitchen. But by learning a few simple knife skills you can slice your own and save money. And it's more fun! Carefully chosen canned, bottled, and boxed foods are another great option. Watch for those tricky additives when you're buying them, but overall, things like nut butters, coconut milk, canned sardines, wild Alaskan salmon, artichokes, and roasted red peppers make great additions to salads. Any packaged foods should contain only a few ingredients, and ones that you recognize such as tomatoes, water, and salt.

Pick a day when you have some free time and do a little planning for your week. If you have any prep work that can be done in advance, this would be the time to do it. Put on your favorite music or podcast, and wash, cut, and store your vegetables, ideally in glass containers, or even freeze them. Make some batches of sauces or dips that will keep for a few days, and create a meal plan for the week. This helps with grocery shopping and with sticking to a budget. Also, try to make at least double the amount of any recipe that you know you'll want to have leftovers of or incorporate into another meal. For example, grass-fed burgers and hand-cut roasted sweet potato fries one night can easily become shepherd's pie the next night.

There are many days you might want to cook without a recipe. In fact, that is what I do over 90 percent of the time for simple, delicious, healthy food. Here are easy ways to cook your veggies and meats:

To Steam Veggies

Pour 250 ml of filtered water into a saucepan and bring it to a boil over high heat. Place a steaming rack or basket over the boiling water. Chop your vegetables and place them in the steamer, cover, and let them cook for 4 to 8 minutes, depending on the denseness of the vegetable.

To Blanch Veggies

Simply submerge your vegetables in boiling water for 1 to 3 minutes, depending on the vegetable, until partially cooked.

To Sauté Veggies

Add 1 tablespoon of coconut oil, ghee, or expeller-pressed sesame oil to a sauté pan. After the oil is hot, add the vegetables, cooking them for 1 to 2 minutes. Dense and somewhat tough vegetables such as cauliflower will need a little longer.

To Griddle Veggies

Heat a griddle pan or light a barbecue and brush with a small amount of olive oil. Place the vegetables in the pan or on the barbeque rack and cook, turning once, until browned.

To Roast Veggies

Preheat the oven to 220°C/425°F/Gas 7. Toss the vegetables with olive oil, butter, or coconut oil, and season with sea salt and pepper. Arrange in a layer on a baking sheet and roast until crispy and tender. Times will vary depending on the vegetable.

To Sauté, Grill, or Roast Meats

Follow the same instructions for veggies, but always use a meat thermometer to assess the internal temperature, inserting it in the thickest part of the meat for accuracy. The following guide provides temperatures at which different meats are considered done.

> Steak: 55 to 57°C/130°F to 135°F for medium rare;
>   60 to 63°C/140°F to 145°F for medium
> Fish: 63°C/145°F
> Chicken: 70°C to 74°C/160°F to 165°F
> Ground beef: 74°C/165°F

TIP 5: HOW TO EAT OUTSIDE THE HOME

If you're invited to a party, have no fear; there are ways to enjoy yourself while staying on track with the plan. First things first, never skip meals. If you feel nervous about the food being served, eat before you arrive so you feel satiated and confident about staying away from junk foods. When people ask me why I am not indulging at a party, I tell them that I'm there for the people, not the food. No one argues with that, and no one can possibly feel insulted by it!

Once you arrive, find the vegetables and dips (as there is almost always at least one of these at every gathering), so if you want to munch on something, you have some pretty healthy options. Volunteering to bring something to every gathering you attend is a surefire way to guarantee there's food you can eat. There are plenty of dips and sides in this book that everyone can enjoy (beginning on page 88). Try your best to avoid alcohol, as it's toxic and sugary and can lead you down a slippery slope of bad choices. Instead, bring or ask for sparkling water with lemon or lime. After your three-week program, you can enjoy your favorite drink from time to time.

Eating at a restaurant is a bit more manageable, as most restaurants are very accommodating to dietary needs. If possible, try to choose the restaurant yourself instead of leaving it up to someone else. That way you can control the types of foods you'll be enjoying. When I go to a restaurant with questionable main courses, I focus on the side dishes. There are often plenty of vegetable options, and there's nothing wrong with getting several sides as your main. You can always ask for a basic chicken or fish dish, or salad with a side of avocado, topped with olive oil and vinegar instead of sugary, creamy dressings. The most important piece of advice: do the best you can and focus on the company you are with, not the food.

TIP 6: HOW TO EAT WITH KIDS

Studies show the family that eats together stays together. Given the opportunity, most kids love to play in the kitchen and are always open to trying new foods as a family. Picky eaters are definitely out there, but keep in mind that it sometimes takes kids a few times of trying something new before they decide whether or not they like it. Also keep in mind that making a big deal out of a picky eater's refusal of a particular food only makes it more likely to occur. No drama. Choose your battles and let kids develop their own palates without stress.

Make mealtime a pleasant, relaxed, joyful experience (good for digestion!) and involve your kids in the cooking process. When they are able to help create a meal, they are more likely to eat it. Food should not be used for punishment or reward. This creates a dangerous emotional relationship with food that can carry into adulthood.

Also, set realistic boundaries about food choices and mealtimes. If you want to raise a healthy eater, my recommendation is not to create separate meals for the kids and adults. Once children are old enough to chew solids, expose them to a variety of foods, including the foods that you eat every day. As long as the meal or food is not super spicy, kids should generally be eating all the healthy and varied foods their parents eat, even when eating out. In Japan, kids eat raw fish, and in parts of Africa kids eat reptiles, not chicken nuggets or macaroni and cheese.

If your child has a sophisticated palate, he or she might enjoy all the meals in this book, but the following are sure to be winners with all kids:*

Breakfast

Walnut Pancakes with Blueberries (page 82)
Strawberry-Mint Chia Pudding (page 87)
Creamy Strawberry and Greens Smoothie (page 61)
Banana-Raspberry-Coconut Smoothie (page 65)

Snacks, Sides, Soups

Deviled Eggs (page 102)
Classic Guacamole (page 93)
Sweet Potato Soup with Coconut and Ginger (page 136)

---

* Be aware of allergens. Many of these recipes contain coconut, nuts, and nut milk.

Lunch or Dinner

Turkey Burgers with Peppers and Onions (page 220)
"Spaghetti" and Meatballs with Tomato Sauce (page 226)
Tempeh, Vegetable, and Kelp Noodle Stir-Fry (page 171)

Dessert

Raspberry-Coconut Ice Cream (page 262)
Spiced Sweet Potato Quick Bread (page 251)
No-Bake Walnut Brownies (page 259)

TIP 7: HOW TO SNACK

The number one thing that can derail your plans is getting caught in a food emergency. When your blood sugar drops, everything, even junk food, can start to look like a good option. Thinking that you can use willpower to maneuver your way out of these situations is not realistic. You need to be prepared for moments like this, especially when you're away from your healthy home base. Snacking is perfectly fine on this program, and even though you might not need snacks because increased fat cuts cravings, I still recommend keeping certain foods on hand in case of an emergency.

The key to smart snacking is to stick to protein, fats, or low-glycemic carbs. The reason this works is because sugary processed carbs are addictive, and we don't know when to stop eating them, but fats and proteins are satiating, and when you've had enough, your body tells you instantly. Do you ever find yourself overeating broccoli? I didn't think so. We've included plenty of snack recipes starting on page 88, but if you are looking for items to purchase and take on the go, these are my recommendations:

- Canned wild salmon or sardines
- Jerky (bison, grass-fed beef, salmon, or turkey)
- Nuts and seeds (almonds, walnuts, pecans, macadamia nuts, and pumpkin seeds)

- Nut butter, single-serving sachets (almond, pecan, macadamia)
- Coconut butter (you can buy it in convenient single-serving sachets)

For short trips and to take to the office or school:

- Hard-boiled omega-3 eggs
- Cut-up carrots, cucumbers, peppers, and celery in ziplock baggies (pair with guacamole)
- 75 g mixed berries in a small bag
- Sometimes I love to cut open an avocado, sprinkle a little salt or wheat-free tamari or balsamic vinegar on top of it, and eat it with a spoon.

My favorite snack pack includes canned wild salmon, grass-fed jerky, nuts and seeds, and almond butter squeeze packs. When you're traveling or running out of time, this snack pack will prevent you from running into a food emergency.

TIP 8: HOW TO SWAP GOOD FOR BAD

Cravings for your old favorites may pop up from time to time, but there are always healthier alternatives. So try these instead of those.

Instead of	Try
Bread	Spiced Sweet Potato Quick Bread (page 251)
Crisps	Nuts (almonds, cashews, macadamia nuts, etc.) Dehydrated or roasted veggies such as kale, carrots, courgettes
Fizzy drinks	Sparkling water with a little bit of lemon or lime
Pasta	Kelp noodles, courgette noodles, spaghetti squash

(continued)

Instead of	Try
Yogurt	Strawberry-Mint Chia Pudding (page 87), coconut yogurt
Sweets	Mixed berries
Mashed potatoes	Butternut squash, sweet potato mash, cauliflower mash
Cheese	Nutritional yeast
Peanut butter	Almond butter, cashew butter, coconut butter

TIP 9: HOW TO DEAL WITH YOUR HEALING CRISIS

It is not uncommon for the body to have a strong reaction when you stop feeding it the processed foods and chemicals it is accustomed to. This is called a healing crisis or a detox crisis.

Food companies have chemically engineered their foods to be biologically addictive, and the result is that many people are hooked on processed junk food. Ridding your system of these toxic foods can cause some uncomfortable reactions, such as achy, flu-like feelings, irritability, nausea, headaches, sleep difficulties, and constipation. The good news is that these symptoms usually pass within forty-eight hours. So first and foremost, give your body time to adjust. If possible, start the twenty-one-day plan on a weekend or when you have some time off to lay a bit lower than usual for a day or two if you need to.

A strong negative reaction to a cleanse or detox is more common with calorie-restrictive programs such as juice cleanses, so that's why I always recommend food-based programs to avoid detoxing too quickly. Prep days or transition weeks are also helpful to get your body adjusted to the types of foods you'll be eating. If the *Eat Fat, Get Thin* Plan is drastically different from your normal diet, I recommend giving yourself a few days to experiment with the approved foods and get used to things slowly, before adding in supplements.

Another way to ease healing-crisis symptoms is to increase circulation and flush the toxins out of your body by going for a walk outside, taking a sauna, or getting a massage. It's very important to make sure your bowels are moving. If you're backed up, toxins will remain in the body and you'll feel pretty awful. To combat constipation, first and foremost, stay hydrated. Try sprinkling ground flaxseeds into your salads or smoothies. Magnesium citrate also helps with bowels, sleep, and stress. If none of those strategies work, you can take a herbal laxative such as cascara, senna, or rhubarb. De-stress however possible, because stress is incredibly constipating.

Other options to ease your detox include getting plenty of rest. Make your bedroom a tranquil haven and your bed a place for sleep or romance only. Try to avoid screen time and eating for at least one to two hours before bed.

Going low-carb very quickly can cause a drop in energy for some people. If you feel fatigued for more than a few days, contact one of our coaches at www.drhyman.com. Most of the time, adding salt or E-lyte electrolytes can help as you are getting off the carbs. When you drop your insulin level you will drop a lot of retained fluid and salt along with it, so adding more salt helps prevent you from feeling dizzy and weak.

If your detox symptoms persist for a longer period of time, it may mean that something deeper is going on, and in that case I recommend the help of a Functional Medicine practitioner (page 12), but one to three days of adjustment is common for most people.

4

Transitioning to the Pegan Diet

After twenty-one days, you have the option of staying on the *Eat Fat, Get Thin* Plan or transitioning to what I call the Pegan Diet. After years of experimenting with different diets (vegan, vegetarian, Paleo, low-fat, low-carb) and seeing thousands of patients, I've finally landed on this one. It has left me feeling better than ever and has transformed the lives of people all over the world.

What is Pegan? Well, a Pegan Diet combines the best of the Paleo and vegan diets, which have a lot more in common than you might think. A healthy vegan diet and a healthy Paleo diet place an emphasis on real, whole, fresh food that is sustainably raised and is rich in vitamins, minerals, and phytonutrients, while being low in sugar, refined carbs, and processed foods and ingredients. Essentially, the Pegan Diet is all about eating real food.

In order to determine whether or not you should transition, I recommend heading over to www.eatfatgetthin.com/resources and taking the recommended quizzes, tests, and measurements before and after the twenty-one days. There are two quizzes in particular (the Feel Like Crap Quiz and the Carbohydrate Intolerance Quiz) that will show you your toxicity levels before you start the program and after. I highly recommend taking these quizzes so that you can monitor your progress and decide whether or not to stay on the *Eat Fat, Get Thin* Plan or transition.

Here are the steps to transitioning to a Pegan Diet:

1. Add in beans and gluten-free grains such as black rice, quinoa, and buckwheat in moderation. See what works for your unique body.

For some, these foods might cause inflammation, a spike in insulin and blood sugar, and digestive issues. So it's best to test these foods out slowly to see how your body reacts to them. Do you feel good or do you feel bloated? Does your skin break out? How are your energy levels? Does any sort of negative reaction follow the consumption of these foods?

2. Continue to eat the right fats. Stay away from inflammatory (processed vegetable) fats and continue to focus on the good fats, such as nuts and seeds, wild fatty fish, avocados, and coconut oil.

3. Eat mostly plants—plenty of low-glycemic vegetables and fruits. These should make up 75 percent of your diet and your plate.

4. Power up with protein. Again, protein is essential for muscle synthesis and appetite control, and it speeds up your metabolism.

5. Stay away from dairy (except for grass-fed butter), because it's inflammatory and filled with hormones.

6. Stay away from gluten. If you are not gluten sensitive, then consider it an occasional treat. Try small amounts of non–gluten grains such as black rice, quinoa, and buckwheat.

7. Continue with the daily supplements and thirty minutes of movement (that you find enjoyable) each day.

8. I'll let you in on a little secret. I don't eat a perfect diet 100 percent of the time. When traveling or socializing, we're all occasionally tempted with "junk" foods. Think of sugar and flour as recreational drugs. Once you've achieved all of your health goals and weight-loss goals, you can indulge in these "recreational treats" occasionally without guilt. (Eating these foods and then punishing yourself with guilt is dangerous for your emotional and physical health, so make sure you skip the self-reproach.) I've included some of my favorite dessert recipes for just these occasions (page 250).

You'll see Pegan recipes throughout this book. Just look for "Pegan Diet" underneath the recipe title. If you're on the twenty-one-day *Eat Fat, Get Thin* Plan, skip these recipes for now.

The Pegan Diet Food Pyramid

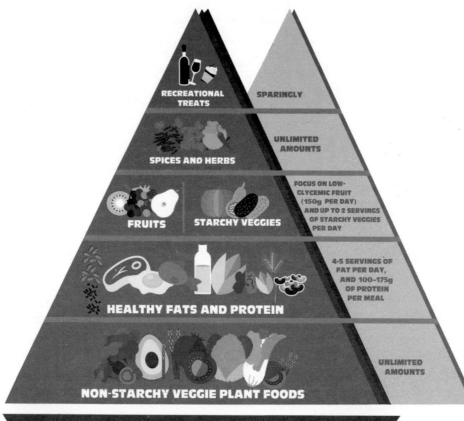

RECREATIONAL TREATS — SPARINGLY

SPICES AND HERBS — UNLIMITED AMOUNTS

FRUITS | STARCHY VEGGIES — FOCUS ON LOW-GLYCEMIC FRUIT (150g PER DAY) AND UP TO 2 SERVINGS OF STARCHY VEGGIES PER DAY

HEALTHY FATS AND PROTEIN — 4-5 SERVINGS OF FAT PER DAY, AND 100–175g OF PROTEIN PER MEAL

NON-STARCHY VEGGIE PLANT FOODS — UNLIMITED AMOUNTS

DR. MARK HYMAN'S PEGAN FOOD PYRAMID

PART II

THE RECIPES

We have the power to transform our food industry and the health of the world. This transformation starts with you and what you put into your shopping carts, stock your home with, and serve on your kitchen table. It starts with what you eat every single day.

I believe we can vote with our dollars. Every time we purchase packaged, processed, GMO foods, we vote to keep ourselves sick and our planet sick. We also tell the corporations that's what we want. Every time we fill our kitchens with beautiful, real, whole, fresh foods and support our small local farms, we vote to keep ourselves and our planet healthy, and we send a loud and clear message to those same corporations.

Reconnecting with cooking and my kitchen has been one of the most transformative experiences of my life. Cooking has brought my family closer together. It has made me healthier, given me more energy and new goals, and created a new joy that I look forward to every mealtime. I believe that everyone is capable of achieving this joy by using food as medicine.

I am so thrilled to have teamed up with my friend Chef Frank Giglio to present these mouthwatering yet simple recipes that I hope will bring you as much pleasure as they bring me. Now you have all the tools you need. Let's get cooking!

Remember that all recipes that say "Pegan Diet" underneath the title are to be used after the twenty-one-day plan. All other recipes can be enjoyed at any time.

5

Smoothies and Beverages

BASIC NUT MILK

Shop-bought nut milks often contain fillers and synthetic vitamins, so I recommend that you make your own. It's much easier than you might think. Just remember to soak the nuts overnight to soften them so that they blend more easily. Soaking also unlocks nutrients, making them easier to absorb and digest.

Makes: 1 litre (strained)
Prep time: 2 minutes, plus 12 to 24 hours for soaking

- 50 g raw almonds (or 100 g raw walnuts, or 135 g raw hazelnuts or Brazil nuts)
- 1 litre filtered water, plus extra for soaking

Place the nuts in a glass container and add enough filtered water to cover the almonds by about 5 cm. Cover and refrigerate for at least 12 hours, or for up to 24 hours.

Drain the nuts. Combine the nuts and measured water in a blender. Begin blending on a low speed, slowly increasing to high, then blend on high speed for 1 to 1½ minutes.

You can use the nut milk as is, or, for a smoother consistency, strain the mixture through a nut-milk bag (available at healthfood stores and online) into a large bowl; squeeze the bag to extract as much milk as possible from the pulp.

Transfer the nut milk to an airtight container and refrigerate for up to 3 days. Stir well or shake before using.

Nutritional analysis per serving (250ml strained almond milk): *Calories: 128, Fat: 11.2 g, Saturated Fat: 0.8 g, Cholesterol: 0 mg, Fiber: 2.4 g, Protein: 4.8 g, Carbohydrates: 4.8 g, Sodium: 0 mg*

Coconut Milk

Coconut milk is my favorite dairy-free alternative, especially for creating delicious smoothies and curries. It contains MCT oils (page 27), a form of fat that has many benefits, among them supporting heart health and helping to build muscle. Full-fat coconut milk straight from the can is often too thick for smoothies, so if you're looking for a lighter flavor and consistency, try this recipe.

Makes: 1 litre
Prep time: 5 minutes

- 1 x 400 ml can full-fat coconut milk
- 550 ml filtered water

Combine the coconut milk and filtered water in a glass container. Stir until well blended, or cover with a tight-fitting lid and shake vigorously. Refrigerate, covered, for up to 5 days.

Nutritional analysis per serving (250 ml): *Calories: 202, Fat: 20 g, Saturated Fat: 19 g, Cholesterol: 0 mg, Fiber: 0 g, Protein: 0 g, Carbohydrates: 3 g, Sodium: 25 mg*

Coconut-Acai Smoothie

PEGAN DIET

Often considered a superfood, acai berries are known for their antioxidant benefits. Acai bowls—a purée of the berries topped with an assortment of fruits and nuts—have become popular breakfast meals. In this recipe, the frozen acai purée is blended with coconut to create a rich, flavorful, nutrient-dense smoothie.

Serves: 1
Prep time: 5 minutes

- 90 g frozen acai, cut into small chunks
- 2 tablespoons chopped raw shelled pistachios
- 1 date, pitted
- 2 teaspoons fresh lemon juice
- 300 ml Coconut Milk (page 55)
- ½ teaspoon vanilla powder

Combine all the ingredients in a blender and blend on high speed until smooth and creamy, about 45 seconds. Drink immediately.

Nutritional analysis per serving: Calories: 336, Fat: 17 g, Saturated Fat: 7 g, Cholesterol: 5 mg, Fiber: 6 g, Protein: 6 g, Carbohydrates: 44 g, Sodium: 15 mg

Mango-Coconut Smoothie

PEGAN DIET

This tropical-flavored smoothie is one of my go-to blends, especially in the summer. It's enhanced with nutrient- and-protein-rich hemp seeds, and with creamy coconut butter, making it a satisfying breakfast choice.

Serves: 1
Prep time: 5 minutes

- 165 g frozen mango chunks
- 375 ml coconut water (or unsweetened nut milk or filtered water)
- 2 tablespoons hemp seeds
- 2 tablespoons coconut butter

Combine all the ingredients in a blender and blend on high speed until smooth and creamy, about 45 seconds. Drink immediately.

Nutritional analysis per serving: *Calories: 562, Fat: 30 g, Saturated Fat: 18 g, Cholesterol: 0 mg, Fiber: 12 g, Protein: 11 g, Carbohydrates: 76 g, Sodium: 111 mg*

Mixed Berry-Coconut Smoothie

Coconut milk is a nutritious and creamy source of high-quality fat, making it the perfect choice for satisfying smoothies like this one. This quick and easy smoothie made with frozen berries is an excellent choice for breakfast or a snack. For added richness, freeze coconut milk in an ice-cube tray and use the frozen cubes in place of regular ice cubes.

Serves: 1
Prep time: 5 minutes

- 225g frozen mixed berries
- 250 ml full-fat coconut milk, chilled
- 8 ice cubes
- 1 teaspoon ground cinnamon
- ½ teaspoon alcohol- and gluten-free pure vanilla extract (or ¼ teaspoon unsweetened vanilla powder)
- grated zest of 1 lemon

Combine all the ingredients in a blender and blend on high speed until smooth and creamy, about 45 seconds. Drink immediately.

Nutritional analysis per serving: *Calories: 327, Fat: 24 g, Saturated Fat: 22 g, Cholesterol: 0 mg, Fiber: 4 g, Protein: 1 g, Carbohydrates: 24 g, Sodium: 47 mg*

CHERRY BOMB SMOOTHIE

PEGAN DIET

Talk about an antioxidant powerhouse! This morning beverage includes a treble dose of healing spices: cinnamon, nutmeg, and ginger. Combined with fatty hazelnuts and antioxidants from cherries, this smoothie will jump-start your day in just the right way.

Serves: 1
Prep time: 5 minutes

- 375 ml unsweetened Hazelnut Milk (page 54)
- 120 g frozen pitted sweet cherries
- ½ teaspoon ground cinnamon
- ½ teaspoon freshly grated nutmeg
- ½ teaspoon ground ginger
- ½ teaspoon alcohol- and gluten-free pure vanilla extract (or ¼ teaspoon unsweetened vanilla powder)
- 1 tablespoon coconut butter

Combine all the ingredients in a blender and blend on high speed until smooth and creamy, about 45 seconds. Drink immediately.

Nutritional analysis per serving: *Calories: 479, Fat: 21 g, Saturated Fat: 8 g, Cholesterol: 0 mg, Fiber: 5 g, Protein: 8 g, Carbohydrates: 68 g, Sodium: 6 mg*

Cherry-Hemp Smoothie

PEGAN DIET

Hemp seeds are a great source of protein, magnesium, zinc, iron, and phosphorus. Needless to say, they are an excellent addition to your diet and are easy to incorporate into smoothies and salads. This five-ingredient smoothie is super-easy to whip together first thing in the morning or after a workout.

Serves: 1
Prep time: 5 minutes

- 375 ml unsweetened Almond Milk (page 54)
- 75 g frozen pitted sweet cherries
- 2 tablespoons hemp seeds
- 1 tablespoon hemp oil
- ½ teaspoon ground ginger

Combine all the ingredients in a blender and blend on high speed until smooth and creamy, about 45 seconds. Drink immediately.

Nutritional analysis per serving: *Calories: 387, Fat: 25 g, Saturated Fat: 2 g, Cholesterol: 0 mg, Fiber: 5 g, Protein: 8 g, Carbohydrates: 29 g, Sodium: 2 mg*

CREAMY STRAWBERRY AND GREENS SMOOTHIE

Rocket is one of the best nutrient–dense leafy greens. It's a great source of phytochemicals and antioxidants, which have been known to combat cancer. Throwing a handful of greens into your smoothie is an easy way to get more nutrients into your diet.

Serves: 1
Prep time: 5 minutes

- 375 ml unsweetened Hazelnut or Almond Milk (page 54)
- ½ avocado, stoned and peeled
- 150 g frozen strawberries
- 1 handful baby rocket leaves
- 1 tablespoon coconut oil, melted

Combine all the ingredients in a blender and blend on high speed until smooth and creamy, about 45 seconds. Drink immediately.

Nutritional analysis per serving: *Calories: 544, Fat: 31 g, Saturated Fat: 15 g, Cholesterol: 0 mg, Fiber: 21 g, Protein: 9 g, Carbohydrates: 42 g, Sodium: 248 mg*

Omega-3 Green Smoothie

Fats + protein + slow carbs is my go-to formula for creating meals that keep me satisfied for hours. This smoothie has that combination, and every single ingredient contains powerful nutrition that will leave you feeling vibrant. I usually start my day with this blend or some variation of it.

Serves: 1
Prep time: 5 minutes

- 375 ml coconut water, chilled
- 1 tablespoon hemp oil
- 1 tablespoon chia seeds
- 150 g frozen strawberries or raspberries
- ½ avocado, stoned and peeled
- 1 large handful baby spinach
- 1 tablespoon toasted shredded coconut, for garnish (optional)

Combine all the ingredients in a blender and blend on high speed until smooth and creamy, about 45 seconds. Top with the toasted coconut, if using, and drink immediately.

Nutritional analysis per serving: *Calories: 530, Fat: 34 g, Saturated Fat: 6 g, Cholesterol: 0 mg, Fiber: 22 g, Protein: 7 g, Carbohydrates: 41 g, Sodium: 368 mg*

Minted Green Smoothie with Raspberries

If you're looking to pack a lot of nutrition into a quick, portable meal, look no further than green smoothies. They're perfect for kids who don't like the taste of greens. Here, peppermint tea imparts a fresh, herbal note.

Serves: 1
Prep time: 5 minutes, plus steeping and cooling time

- 1 peppermint teabag
- 150 g frozen raspberries
- 2 handfuls baby spinach
- 4 ice cubes
- 2 tablespoons hemp seeds
- 1 tablespoon MCT oil (available online)

Place the teabag in a 300-ml heatproof glass container and pour in 275 ml boiling water. Cover and steep for 10 minutes, then remove and discard the bag. Refrigerate the tea until cold.

Combine the chilled tea, raspberries, spinach, ice, hemp seeds, and oil in a blender and blend on high speed until smooth and creamy, about 45 seconds. Drink immediately.

Nutritional analysis per serving: *Calories: 395, Fat: 25 g, Saturated Fat: 15 g, Cholesterol: 0 mg, Fiber: 9 g, Protein: 8 g, Carbohydrates: 19 g, Sodium: 11 mg*

Peachy Green Smoothie

PEGAN DIET

A complete protein, spirulina is high in chlorophyll, B vitamins, and an assortment of minerals. Don't let the blue-green color scare you off! This unique smoothie will surprise you with its delicious flavor.

Serves: 1
Prep time: 5 minutes

- 500 ml unsweetened Almond Milk (page 54), chilled
- 150 g frozen or canned sliced peaches
- 2 tablespoons almond butter
- 1 tablespoon chia seeds
- 2 teaspoons spirulina

Combine all the ingredients in a blender and blend on high speed until smooth and creamy, about 45 seconds. Drink immediately.

Nutritional analysis per serving: *Calories: 441, Fat: 28 g, Saturated Fat: 2 g, Cholesterol: 0 mg, Fiber: 10 g, Protein: 12 g, Carbohydrates: 40 g, Sodium: 379 mg*

Banana-Raspberry-Coconut Smoothie

PEGAN DIET

I think of this smoothie as a drinkable treat. The frozen banana creates a creamy texture that kids will love. As a bonus, the drink is filled with delicious and nutritious high–quality fats.

Serves: 1
Prep time: 5 minutes

- 250 ml coconut water (or filtered water), chilled
- 1 banana, peeled and frozen
- 120 g frozen raspberries
- 2 tablespoons coconut butter
- 1 tablespoon coconut oil
- 60 g baby spinach

Combine all the ingredients in a blender and blend on high speed until smooth and creamy, about 45 seconds. Drink immediately.

Nutritional analysis per serving: *Calories: 625, Fat: 36 g, Saturated Fat: 30 g, Cholesterol: 0 mg, Fiber: 26 g, Protein: 5 g, Carbohydrates: 48 g, Sodium: 248 mg*

Chocolate-Raspberry Smoothie

The classic combination of chocolate and raspberry makes for a double whammy of antioxidants! (Cacao contains large amounts of *both* antioxidants and magnesium.) A little touch of ghee boosts the fat content and enhances this delectable treat of a smoothie.

Serves: 1
Prep time: 5 minutes

- 375 ml unsweetened Nut Milk (page 54), chilled
- 120 g frozen raspberries
- 1 heaped tablespoon cacao powder
- 1 tablespoon Ghee (page 279)
- 2 dates, pitted (optional, use during Pegan Diet)
- 1 teaspoon unsweetened vanilla powder

Combine all the ingredients in a blender and blend on high speed until smooth and creamy, about 45 seconds. Drink immediately.

Nutritional analysis per serving: *Calories: 379, Fat: 20 g, Saturated Fat: 9 g, Cholesterol: 0 mg, Fiber: 11 g, Protein: 7 g, Carbohydrates: 50 g, Sodium: 253 mg*

Pumpkin Pie Bulletproof Coffee

It's Bulletproof Coffee with a seasonal twist. Spiked with the superfat MCT, this beverage will warm you up and keep you satisfied for hours.

Serves: 1
Prep time: 10 minutes, including coffee-brewing time

- 375 ml freshly brewed hot coffee
- 1 tablespoon unsalted, grass-fed butter
- 2 teaspoons MCT oil
- 2 teaspoons pumpkin pie spice (a mixture of nutmeg, cinnamon, cloves, ginger, allspice and mace)
- 1 teaspoon alcohol- and gluten-free pure vanilla extract (or ¼ teaspoon unsweetened vanilla powder)
- 1 tablespoon maple syrup (optional)

Combine all the ingredients in a blender and blend on high speed until frothy, about 45 seconds. Drink immediately.

Nutritional analysis per serving: *Calories: 349, Fat: 33 g, Saturated Fat: 24 g, Cholesterol: 61 mg, Fiber: 1 g, Protein: 0 g, Carbohydrates: 18 g, Sodium: 21 mg*

REISHI MUSHROOM-COFFEE ELIXIR

Reishi mushrooms have an array of health benefits, including immune-system support. If you haven't experimented with reishi mushrooms, I highly recommend trying this hot drink—it's a comforting and tasty introduction. Mushroom extracts and capsules are readily available online and at most healthfood stores.

Serves: 1
Prep time: 5 minutes

- 375 m l freshly brewed hot coffee
- 1 tablespoon Ghee (page 279) or coconut oil
- ½ teaspoon alcohol- and gluten-free pure vanilla extract
- 6 x 1000-mg reishi mushroom capsules

Combine the coffee, ghee, and vanilla in a blender. Open each reishi capsule and empty the contents into the blender, discarding the capsules. Blend on high speed until combined, about 30 seconds. Drink immediately.

Nutritional analysis per serving: Calories: 200, Fat: 11 g, Saturated Fat: 7 g, Cholesterol: 30 mg, Fiber: 0 g, Protein: 0 g, Carbohydrates: 0 g, Sodium: 107 mg

6

Eggs and Other Breakfast Dishes

Slow-Fried Eggs with Onion and Basil

By frying eggs over a gentle heat on a bed of onion slices, you can create soft, creamy eggs that taste almost as if they have been poached. Add some fragrant basil and you have an aromatic dish that will wake up the whole family.

Serves: 4
Prep time: 5 minutes
Cook time: 8 minutes

- 3 tablespoons extra-virgin olive oil
- 2 teaspoons unsalted, grass-fed butter
- 1 small red onion, sliced into very thin rounds
- 4 large eggs
- 1 teaspoon sea salt
- ¼ teaspoon freshly ground black pepper
- 10 g fresh basil leaves, torn into small pieces

In 20-cm frying pan, warm 1 tablespoon of the olive oil and the butter over a medium heat until shimmering. Spread out the onion slices in an even layer and cook without stirring until slightly softened, about 2 minutes. Using a metal spatula, flip the onion slices, then crack an egg into each quadrant of the pan, on top of the onion. Cook for 2 minutes, then drizzle the eggs with 1 tablespoon of the remaining olive oil and sprinkle with the salt and pepper. Partially cover the pan and cook until the egg whites are set but the yolks are still soft, 3 to 4 minutes.

Drizzle the eggs with the remaining tablespoon of olive oil. Transfer 1 egg with some of the onion slices to each of 4 plates, sprinkle with basil and serve.

Nutritional analysis per serving: *Calories: 200, Fat: 19 g, Saturated Fat: 5 g, Cholesterol: 190 mg, Fiber: 0 g, Protein: 6 g, Carbohydrates: 1 g, Sodium: 670 mg*

BUTTERY BROCCOLI AND SPINACH WITH FRIED EGGS

This dish is the perfect way to power up before a long day. It includes my favorite combination of greens, fat and protein, and makes for a comforting, hearty breakfast. I recommend cooking the eggs sunny-side up so that the yolks, when broken, act as a sauce for the vegetables.

Serves: 4
Prep time: 15 minutes
Cook time: 15 minutes

- 225 g broccoli, stems peeled and cut into rounds 5 mm thick, florets cut into bite-sized pieces
- 1½ tablespoons Ghee (page 279)
- ½ onion, thinly sliced
- 2 garlic cloves, crushed
- 120 g baby spinach
- ½ teaspoon sea salt
- ¼ teaspoon freshly ground black pepper
- 1 tablespoon unsalted, grass-fed butter
- 4 large eggs
- 2 avocados, stoned, peeled and sliced

Bring 1 litre of filtered water to the boil in a medium saucepan over a high heat, then add the broccoli. Use a spatula to keep it submerged in the water, and cook until tender, 2 to 3 minutes. Using a slotted spoon, transfer the broccoli to a plate.

Warm the ghee in a large sauté pan over a medium–high heat until melted. Add the onion and cook, stirring occasionally, until softened, 3 to 4 minutes. Stir in the garlic and cook until fragrant, about 30 seconds. Add the spinach and the cooked broccoli and stir to incorporate. Sprinkle the salt and the pepper on top and stir to combine. Remove from the heat and cover to keep warm.

Warm the butter in a 20-cm frying pan over a medium heat until foaming. Carefully crack an egg into each quadrant of the pan and cook until the egg whites are fully set but the yolks are still soft, 3 to 4 minutes.

(For over a easy eggs, use a metal spatula to gently flip each egg and cook for 1 minute.)

Divide the vegetable mixture equally between 4 plates and top each portion with an egg. Garnish with the avocado slices and serve.

Nutritional analysis per serving: Calories: 290, Fat: 23 g, Saturated Fat: 7 g, Cholesterol: 187 mg, Fiber: 11 g, Protein: 12 g, Carbohydrates: 15 g, Sodium: 721 mg

POACHED EGGS WITH HOLLANDAISE

Hollandaise gets an upgrade, with ghee replacing the butter. Serve asparagus or sautéed spinach alongside the eggs and hollandaise for a perfect brunch.

Serves: 4
Prep time: 10 minutes
Cook time: 30 minutes

- 8 large eggs, plus 3 yolks
- 175 g Ghee (page 279), melted and kept warm
- ½ teaspoon sea salt
- 2 teaspoons fresh lemon juice
- generous pinch of cayenne pepper
- 2 tablespoons apple cider vinegar

Pour a 2.5-cm depth of water into a saucepan, bring to a simmer over a medium heat, then reduce the heat to low.

Place the egg yolks in a medium heatproof bowl, add 1 teaspoon cold water and whisk until the yolks lighten in color, 1 to 2 minutes. Set the bowl over the pan of simmering water (making sure the bottom of the bowl doesn't touch the water) and whisk constantly until the mixture is thick enough to coat the back of a spoon, 3 to 5 minutes.

Remove the bowl from the pan and gradually whisk in the warm ghee, drop by drop to start, then increasing to a slow but steady stream. Add the salt, lemon juice and cayenne and whisk to combine. Place the bowl back over the simmering water occasionally so that the hollandaise stays warm until you are ready to serve, but be careful not to let it overheat or the sauce will split.

Pour a 5-cm depth of filtered water into a 2-litre saucepan and bring to a simmer over a medium heat. Stir in the vinegar. Crack 1 egg at a time into a ramekin or teacup, then carefully slide it into the water. Repeat with the remaining eggs, then let them all cook undisturbed until the whites are just set but the yolks are still soft, 3 to 4 minutes.

Using a slotted spoon, place 2 poached eggs on each serving plate. Drizzle warm hollandaise over the top and serve.

Nutritional analysis per serving: *Calories: 588, Fat: 58 g, Saturated Fat: 31 g, Cholesterol: 508 mg, Fiber: 0 g, Protein: 14 g, Carbohydrates: 1 g, Sodium: 426 mg*

EGGS BAKED ON PORTOBELLO MUSHROOMS

This is a fun recipe to make for breakfast or brunch guests. As they bake, the meaty mushroom caps soften and absorb the herby pesto, so they're flavored throughout. Make sure not to overcook the eggs because the soft yolks act as a sauce for the mushrooms.

Serves: 4
Prep time: 20 minutes
Cook time: 15 minutes

- 4 large portobello mushrooms
- 2 tablespoons extra-virgin olive oil
- 125 ml Rocket Pesto (page 269)
- 4 large eggs
- 12 cherry tomatoes, cut in half

Preheat the oven to 180°C/350°F/Gas 4.

Remove and discard the stems from the mushrooms. Using a spoon, gently scrape away the gills from the underside of the mushroom caps. If the caps don't sit stably with the stemmed sides facing up, trim the rounded sides so that they do.

Place the caps stemmed-side up in a 33 x 23-cm baking dish and drizzle them with the olive oil. Spread 2 tablespoons of the pesto on each cap, then carefully crack an egg on top. Place 6 cherry tomato halves around each egg. Bake until the egg whites have set but the yolks are still a bit runny, 6 to 8 minutes.

Carefully transfer each egg-topped mushroom to a plate and serve.

Nutritional analysis per serving: *Calories: 209, Fat: 16 g, Saturated Fat: 3 g, Cholesterol: 187 mg, Fiber: 3 g, Protein: 9 g, Carbohydrates: 6 g, Sodium: 158 mg*

ITALIAN BREAKFAST SCRAMBLE

Here's a delicious breakfast to enjoy in the summer, when tomatoes and cour-gettes are at the height of their season. Basil is rich in potassium and a good source of iron and vitamins A, C and K. The addition of this powerful, aro-matic herb will make you feel as though you're holidaying in Italy.

Serves: 4
Prep time: 15 minutes
Cook time: 10 minutes

- 4 large eggs
- 1 teaspoon sea salt
- ¼ teaspoon freshly ground black pepper
- 2 tablespoons extra-virgin olive oil
- 1 courgette, finely diced
- 1 small red onion, finely diced
- 2 garlic cloves, thinly sliced
- 8 cherry tomatoes, cut in half
- 10 g julienned fresh basil
- 1 tablespoon unsalted, grass-fed butter, at room temperature

Put the eggs, salt and pepper in a bowl and whisk together.

Warm the olive oil in a large nonstick frying pan over a medium heat until shimmering. Add the courgette and onion and cook, stirring occa-sionally, until softened, 2 to 3 minutes. Stir in the garlic and cook until fragrant, about 1 minute. Add the tomatoes and cook just until heated through, 3 to 4 minutes.

Pour in the eggs and, using a wooden spoon, stir until they form soft curds, about 3 minutes. Remove from the heat, fold in the basil and but-ter, and serve.

Nutritional analysis per serving: *Calories: 392, Fat: 15 g, Saturated Fat: 4 g, Cholesterol: 193 mg, Fiber: 4 g, Protein: 16 g, Carbohydrates: 53 g, Sodium: 533 mg*

SPICY EGG SCRAMBLE WITH TOMATO AND AVOCADO

Liven up your egg breakfast with this spicy twist on basic scrambled eggs. Chilies contain capsaicin, an anti–inflammatory substance that has been shown to promote healthy weight loss. Feel free to turn up the heat or turn it down by using more or less chili.

Serves: 4
Prep time: 10 minutes
Cook time: 10 minutes

- 8 large eggs
- ¼ teaspoon sea salt
- ½ teaspoon freshly ground black pepper
- 2 tablespoons coconut oil
- 1 large red onion, thinly sliced
- 1 jalapeño chili, sliced into thin rounds
- 1 large tomato, roughly chopped
- 1 avocado, stoned, peeled and sliced
- 4 g fresh coriander leaves, roughly chopped

Put the eggs, salt and pepper in a bowl and whisk together.

Warm the coconut oil in a large nonstick frying pan over a medium heat until shimmering. Add the onion and chili and cook, stirring occasionally, until softened, 4 to 5 minutes. Pour in the eggs and, using a wooden spoon, stir until they form soft curds, about 3 minutes.

Divide the eggs between 4 plates. Top with some tomato, avocado slices and coriander and serve.

Nutritional analysis per serving: *Calories: 247, Fat: 21 g, Saturated Fat: 8 g, Cholesterol: 370 mg, Fiber: 4 g, Protein: 14 g, Carbohydrates: 11 g, Sodium: 293 mg*

MUSHROOM AND EGG SCRAMBLE

Mushrooms bring a meaty, earthy quality to any dish. In this recipe, I opt for cremini mushrooms, or baby portobellos as they are sometimes called. If you're a fan of fungi, try experimenting with other varieties, such as oyster and shiitake, or even with more unusual mushrooms such as black trumpet or lion's mane.

Serves: 4
Prep time: 10 minutes
Cook time: 10 minutes

- 8 large eggs
- 3 spring onions, thinly sliced
- 1 teaspoon sea salt
- 2 tablespoons coconut oil
- 350 g cremini mushrooms, thinly sliced
- 2 avocados, stoned, peeled and diced

Put the eggs, spring onions and salt in a bowl and whisk together.

Warm the coconut oil in a large frying pan over a medium–high heat until melted. Add the mushrooms and cook, stirring frequently, until softened and lightly browned, about 3 minutes. Pour in the eggs and, using a wooden spoon, stir until they form soft curds, 2 to 3 minutes.

Divide the scramble between 4 plates. Top with the diced avocados and serve.

Nutritional analysis per serving: *Calories: 296, Fat: 25 g, Saturated Fat: 10 g, Cholesterol: 185 mg, Fiber: 9 g, Protein: 9 g, Carbohydrates: 13 g, Sodium: 508 mg*

SMOKED SALMON AND ASPARAGUS FRITTATA

A frittata is one of my go-to dishes when I want a nutritious, satisfying meal without a lot of time-consuming or labour-intensive cooking.

Serves: 4
Prep time: 15 minutes
Cook time: 35 minutes, plus cooling time

- 8 large eggs
- 125 ml full-fat coconut milk
- 2 tablespoons finely chopped chives
- ½ teaspoon freshly ground black pepper
- 2 tablespoons coconut oil
- 1 onion, chopped
- 2 garlic cloves, crushed
- 1 bunch asparagus, trimmed and cut into 2.5-cm pieces
- 100 g smoked salmon, cut into 5-mm pieces

Preheat the oven to 180°C/350°F/Gas 4. Put the eggs, coconut milk, chives and pepper in a bowl and whisk together.

Warm the coconut oil in a 20-cm ovenproof frying pan over a medium-high heat until shimmering. Add the onion and cook, stirring occasionally, until softened, 2 to 3 minutes. Stir in the garlic and cook until fragrant, about 1 minute. Add the asparagus and cook, stirring occasionally, until slightly softened, 2 to 3 minutes. Stir in the salmon, then pour in the egg mixture. Transfer the pan to the oven and cook until the center of the frittata is firm to the touch and the eggs are fully set (a cocktail stick inserted into the center should come out clean), about 20 minutes.

Allow the frittata to cool for 5 minutes, then carefully run a spatula around the edge and underneath to loosen it from the pan. Slide the frittata onto a plate, cut into 4 wedges and serve.

Nutritional analysis per serving: *Calories: 347, Fat: 26 g, Saturated Fat: 15 g, Cholesterol: 370 mg, Fiber: 3 g, Protein: 22 g, Carbohydrates: 6 g, Sodium: 514 mg*

KIMCHI AND SPINACH FRITTATA

This simple frittata features two very important ingredients: spinach, a vitamin- and mineral-dense supergreen, and kimchi (Korean fermented vegetables), a probiotic-rich food that can improve gut function.

Serves: 4
Prep time: 5 minutes
Cook time: 25 minutes

- 6 large eggs
- 125 ml full-fat coconut milk
- ½ teaspoon sea salt
- ¼ teaspoon freshly ground black pepper
- 1 tablespoon unsalted, grass-fed butter
- 180 g baby spinach
- 75 g drained kimchi, roughly chopped

Preheat the oven to 180°C/350°F/Gas 4.

Put the eggs, coconut milk, salt and pepper in a bowl and whisk together.

Warm the butter in a 20-cm ovenproof frying pan over a medium heat until foaming. Add the spinach and stir until wilted. Pour in the egg mixture, add the kimchi, and stir to evenly distribute. Transfer the pan to the oven and cook until the center of the frittata is firm to the touch and the eggs are fully set (a cocktail stick inserted into the center should come out clean), about 20 minutes.

Allow the frittata to cool for 5 minutes, then carefully run a spatula around the edge and underneath to loosen it from the pan. Slide the frittata onto a plate, cut into 4 wedges and serve hot, warm or at room temperature.

Nutritional analysis per serving: *Calories: 249, Fat: 16 g, Saturated Fat: 9 g, Cholesterol: 285 mg, Fiber: 7 g, Protein: 22 g, Carbohydrates: 14 g, Sodium: 726 mg*

Garlicky Beef and Spinach Frittata

This hearty breakfast is rich in healthy fats from the beef, eggs and ghee. Garlic, known for its anti-inflammatory and medicinal properties, adds a delectable flavor and aroma to the frittata.

Serves: 4
Prep time: 10 minutes
Cook time: 25 minutes, plus cooling time

- 8 large eggs
- 2 teaspoons sea salt
- 2 tablespoons Ghee (page 279)
- 1 large onion, finely diced
- 3 garlic cloves, crushed
- 225 g beef flank steak, cut across the grain into thin strips
- 15 g baby spinach

Preheat the oven to 180°C/350°F/Gas 4.

Put the eggs and salt in a bowl and whisk together.

Warm the ghee in a 20-cm nonstick ovenproof frying pan over a medium heat until melted. Add the onion and cook, stirring occasionally, until softened, 2 to 3 minutes. Stir in the garlic and cook until fragrant, about 1 minute. Stir in the beef and cook until the slices are medium-rare, about 2 minutes. Add the spinach and stir constantly until has wilted. Pour in the eggs and stir to distribute evenly. Transfer the pan to the oven and cook until the center of the frittata is firm to the touch and the eggs are fully set (a cocktail stick inserted into the center should come out clean), about 20 minutes.

Allow the frittata to cool for 5 minutes, then carefully run a spatula around the edge and underneath to loosen it from the pan. Slide the frittata onto a plate, cut into 4 wedges and serve.

Nutritional analysis per serving: *Calories: 667, Fat: 24 g, Saturated Fat: 10 g, Cholesterol: 408 mg, Fiber: 6 g, Protein: 40 g, Carbohydrates: 80 g, Sodium: 1096 mg*

SOUTHWESTERN TOFU SCRAMBLE

This hearty, flavorful scramble can be enjoyed by vegans and omnivores alike.

Serves: 4
Prep time: 20 minutes
Cook time: 15 minutes

- 450 g non-GMO firm tofu
- 2 tablespoons extra-virgin olive oil
- 1 small onion, finely diced
- 1 sweet red pepper, seeded and finely diced
- 1 sweet green pepper, seeded and finely diced
- 1 summer squash, finely diced
- 2 garlic cloves, crushed
- 2 teaspoons chili powder
- 1 teaspoon ground cumin
- 1 teaspoon sea salt
- 1 large tomato, roughly chopped
- 8 g fresh coriander leaves, roughly chopped
- 10 g toasted pumpkin seeds

Use a clean cloth to squeeze any excess water out of the tofu, then use a fork or knife to crumble the tofu into bite-sized pieces.

Warm the olive oil in a large frying pan over a medium-high heat until shimmering. Add the onion, peppers, squash and garlic and cook, stirring occasionally, until the vegetables are slightly softened, about 3 minutes. Stir in the tofu and cook until warmed through, about 3 minutes. Sprinkle in the chili powder, cumin and salt and stir to combine. Add the tomato and cook, stirring occasionally, until it has broken down and any moisture has evaporated, 4 to 5 minutes.

Divide between 4 plates. Top with the coriander and pumpkin seeds and serve.

Nutritional analysis per serving: *Calories: 468, Fat: 16 g, Saturated Fat: 2 g, Cholesterol: 0 mg, Fiber: 9 g, Protein: 24 g, Carbohydrates: 64 g, Sodium: 763 mg*

Walnut Pancakes with Blueberries

Who said that being healthy means giving up pancakes? These delicious breakfast treats are grain-free, sugar-free and dairy-free, so they're completely guilt-free too! The whole family will love them.

Serves: 4
Prep time: 5 minutes
Cook time: 15 minutes

- 6 large eggs
- 375 ml unsweetened Almond Milk (page 54)
- 1 tablespoon fresh lemon juice
- 2 teaspoons alcohol- and gluten-free pure vanilla extract
- 110 g coconut flour
- 130 g arrowroot flour
- 2 teaspoons ground cinnamon
- 1 teaspoon baking powder
- 1 teaspoon bicarbonate of soda
- ½ teaspoon sea salt
- 150 g toasted walnuts, roughly chopped
- coconut oil, for frying
- 150 g blueberries

Whisk the eggs in a large bowl. Add the almond milk, lemon juice and vanilla and whisk until well blended.

Put the coconut flour in a separate bowl, add the arrowroot, cinnamon, baking powder, bicarbonate of soda and salt and mix together. While whisking continuously, add the flour mixture to the egg mixture a tablespoonful at a time. Gently fold in the walnuts.

Warm 1 tablespoon coconut oil in a large frying pan over a medium heat. Meanwhile, measure 65 ml batter into a ladle and note how high it comes. When the pan is hot, ladle the measured batter into the pan to form a 7.5–cm circle, then add as many more circles of batter as will comfortably fit. Cook the pancakes until bubbles appear on the surface, 2 to 3 minutes. Use a metal spatula to flip each pancake and cook for 2 to 3 more minutes. Transfer the pancakes to a wire rack. Add more coconut oil to the pan and repeat to cook the remaining batter.

Divide the pancakes between 4 plates. Top with the blueberries and serve.

Nutritional analysis per serving: Calories: 315, Fat: 15 g, Saturated Fat: 11 g, Cholesterol: 139 mg, Fiber: 11.5 g, Protein: 9 g, Carbohydrates: 35.5 g, Sodium: 293 mg

Buckwheat Porridge

Most people think buckwheat is a grain, but it is actually a seed. I like to use buckwheat not only because it is rich in fiber, but also because it contains protein, can improve digestion, and is a good source of powerful antioxidants. This hearty, nutty-tasting porridge is a great gluten-free alternative to the usual oat variety.

Serves: 4
Prep time: ???
Cook time: 20 minutes

- 165 g buckwheat groats
- 750 ml unsweetened Almond Milk (page 54)
- 1 cinnamon stick
- 1 teaspoon alcohol- and gluten-free pure vanilla extract
- generous pinch of sea salt
- 4 tablespoons maple syrup
- 150 g mixed berries
- 2 tablespoons unsweetened shredded coconut, toasted

Put the buckwheat groats in a saucepan and add the almond milk, cinnamon, vanilla and salt. Cover and cook over a medium heat, stirring occasionally, until the buckwheat is tender and has absorbed the milk, about 20 minutes. Discard the cinnamon stick.

Divide the porridge between 4 bowls. Drizzle each portion with 1 tablespoon of the maple syrup, top equally with the berries, and sprinkle with the toasted coconut. Serve.

Nutritional analysis per serving: Calories: 186, Fat: 5 g, Saturated Fat: 2 g, Cholesterol: 0 mg, Fiber: 4 g, Protein: 3 g, Carbohydrates: 33 g, Sodium: 426 mg

Sprouted Buckwheat Muesli

PEGAN DIET

For those mornings when you're looking for a hearty, egg-free meal, look no further than this muesli. The buckwheat, nuts and seeds in this recipe are soaked for easier digestion. You can tailor the muesli to suit your taste, so try using different nuts and seeds, and even different fruits. Feel free to experiment.

Makes: about 500 g
Prep time: 10 minutes, plus overnight soaking

- 330 g buckwheat groats
- 100 g raw pecans
- 50 g raw walnuts
- 20 g raw pumpkin seeds
- 20 g shelled raw sunflower seeds
- 80 gunsweetened shredded coconut
- 2 crisp, tart apples, grated down to the cores
- 2 teaspoons ground cinnamon
- 1 litre unsweetened Nut Milk (page 54)
- 4 tablespoons maple syrup (optional)

Put the buckwheat groats in a bowl and cover with 1 litre filtered water. Set aside to soak for 2 hours at room temperature.

Drain the buckwheat in a colander and rinse well. Transfer to a shallow container, cover with a clean tea towel and leave to sit at room temperature until the groats begin to sprout, at least 8 hours or even overnight. Rinse and drain well.

While the buckwheat soaks, combine all the nuts and seeds in a bowl. Cover with about 5 cm of filtered water and set aside to soak at room temperature for 2 to 4 hours. Drain and rinse.

Put the sprouted buckwheat in a large bowl, add the soaked nuts and seeds, the coconut, grated apples and cinnamon and stir to combine.

Divide the muesli between 4 serving bowls and pour in 250 ml of the nut milk. Drizzle 1 tablespoon maple syrup, if using, over each portion and serve.

Nutritional analysis per serving (85 g): Calories: 578, Fat: 43 g, Saturated Fat: 13 g, Cholesterol: 0 mg, Fiber: 10 g, Protein: 13 g, Carbohydrates: 43 g, Sodium: 159 mg

STRAWBERRY-MINT CHIA PUDDING

Chia seed pudding is all the rage these days, and it's not hard to see why. Chia is a great source of protein, fiber and fats, and the neutral-tasting seeds absorb water easily and quickly become gelatinous. This is a pudding that's great for breakfast and for taking on the road for a midday snack.

Serves: 1
Prep time: 5 minutes, plus 30 minutes to 12 hours chiling time

- 250 ml unsweetened Almond Milk (page 54)
- 70 g frozen strawberries
- 40 g chia seeds
- ½ teaspoon alcohol- and gluten-free pure vanilla extract
- 2 drops peppermint essential oil
- 70 g fresh strawberries, hulled and sliced
- 1 tablespoon unsweetened coconut flakes

Combine the almond milk and frozen strawberries in a blender and blend on high speed until smooth, about 30 seconds.

Place the chia seeds in a small mixing bowl, then stir in the milk mixture, vanilla and peppermint oil. Cover and refrigerate for at least 30 minutes, or for up to 12 hours.

Top with the sliced fresh strawberries and coconut and serve.

Nutritional analysis per serving: *Calories: 517, Fat: 30 g, Saturated Fat: 17 g, Cholesterol: 0 mg, Fiber: 21 g, Protein: 9 g, Carbohydrates: 42 g, Sodium: 248 mg*

7

Appetizers and Snacks

Coconut-Curry Cashews

Here the spiciness of curry powder is offset by the natural sweetness of raisins. Cashews are one of my favorite nuts and a good source of copper, phosphorus, magnesium, manganese and zinc, making this simple snack a nutritious way to nibble.

Makes: about 350 g
Cook time: 35 minutes

- 70 g raisins
- 275 g raw cashews
- 2 tablespoons unsweetened shredded coconut
- 1 tablespoon curry powder
- 1 teaspoon sea salt

Put the raisins in a small bowl and cover with 175 ml boiling filtered water. Set aside to soak for 30 minutes.

Preheat the oven to 140°C/275°F/Gas 1. Line a baking sheet with baking parchment.

Transfer the raisins and their soaking water to a blender and blend on high speed for about 45 seconds. The purée should have the consistency of a loose paste; if it's watery, pour it into a fine-mesh sieve set over a bowl and let the excess moisture drain off.

Transfer the raisin purée to a bowl, add the cashews, coconut, curry powder and salt and mix until well combined. Spread the mixture on to the prepared baking sheet and bake, stirring every 10 to 15 minutes, until the cashews are golden brown, 25 to 30 minutes.

Allow the cashews to cool completely and serve right away, or store in an airtight container at room temperature for up to 1 month.

Nutritional analysis per serving (70 g): *Calories: 250, Fat: 13 g, Saturated Fat: 7 g, Cholesterol: 0 mg, Fiber: 2 g, Protein: 4 g, Carbohydrates: 34 g, Sodium: 448 mg*

Herb-Roasted Almonds

Nutritious snacks like this one are essential for staying on course with healthful eating while travelling, when at work, or simply when out and about. Almonds are a great source of healthy fats that help keep you feeling full. They also contain powerful prebiotics, especially in the skins, that are food for the friendly bacteria in the gut.

Makes: 175 g
Prep time: 10 minutes
Cook time: 40 minutes

- 450 g raw almonds
- 2 tablespoons extra-virgin olive oil
- 1 tablespoon sea salt
- leaves from a 10-cm rosemary sprig, finely chopped
- leaves from 2 large thyme sprigs, finely chopped
- 1 teaspoon onion powder
- ½ teaspoon garlic powder
- ½ teaspoon ground fennel seed
- ½ teaspoon freshly ground black pepper

Preheat the oven to 140°C/275°F/Gas 1. Line a baking sheet with baking parchment.

Combine all the ingredients in a large bowl and mix well. Spread the almonds in an even layer on the prepared baking sheet and bake, stirring every 15 minutes, until golden brown, 30 to 40 minutes.

Allow the almonds to cool completely and serve right away, or store in an airtight container at room temperature for up to 1 month.

Nutritional analysis per serving (2 tablespoons): *Calories: 178, Fat: 16 g, Saturated Fat: 1 g, Cholesterol: 0 mg, Fiber: 3 g, Protein: 6 g, Carbohydrates: 6 g, Sodium: 420 mg*

Avocado Halves with Spicy Hemp Salt

In this simple recipe, already-delicious avocados get a flavor upgrade with seasoned salt. I like to make a big batch of this seasoning and store it in an airtight container. It's great for sprinkling on salads and can be used in place of regular salt in just about any recipe.

Serves: 4
Prep time: 5 minutes

- 2 tablespoons hemp seeds
- 1 tablespoon nutritional yeast
- 1 teaspoon sea salt
- ½ teaspoon garlic powder
- ¼ teaspoon cayenne pepper
- 4 avocados, halved and stoned

Put all the dry ingredients in a small bowl and stir together.

Sprinkle the hemp salt evenly over the avocado halves. Serve with spoons for scooping the avocado flesh from the skin.

Nutritional analysis per serving: *Calories: 302, Fat: 26 g, Saturated Fat: 4 g, Cholesterol: 0 mg, Fiber: 12 g, Protein: 7 g, Carbohydrates: 19 g, Sodium: 574 mg*

Avocado and Vegetable Salsa

Most dips and salsas that you find at the supermarket are filled with preservatives, so I vote for homemade instead. This way, you're able to monitor what you're putting into your body. Here's a rich, delicious salsa that's also very versatile—serve it with crudités or linseed crackers as a snack or appetizer, or offer it as an accompaniment to fish and other proteins.

Makes: 1 litre
Prep time: 10 minutes

- 3 avocados, stoned, peeled and cut into 1-cm chunks
- 6 cherry tomatoes, cut in half
- 1 sweet red pepper, seeded and finely diced
- 1 celery stick, finely diced
- 2 spring onions, thinly sliced
- 60 g fresh parsley leaves, roughly chopped
- 2 tablespoons hemp seeds
- 2 tablespoons fresh lemon juice
- 3 tablespoons extra-virgin olive oil
- 1 teaspoon sea salt
- ¼ teaspoon freshly ground black pepper

Toss all the ingredients together in a large bowl until well mixed. Serve right away or cover and refrigerate for up to 2 hours.

Nutritional analysis per serving (250 ml): *Calories: 377, Fat: 35 g, Saturated Fat: 5 g, Cholesterol: 0 mg, Fiber: 11 g, Protein: 9 g, Carbohydrates: 16 g, Sodium: 456 mg*

CLASSIC GUACAMOLE

Everyone should have a good recipe for guacamole in their repertoire. There are no surprises here — this is the classic, crowd-pleasing dip.

Makes: about 450 g
Prep time: 10 minutes

- 2 large avocados, halved and stoned
- 1 small onion, finely chopped
- 1 jalapeño chili, seeded and finely chopped
- 5 g fresh coriander leaves, roughly chopped
- 1 teaspoon sea salt
- juice of 1 lime, plus more if needed
- 1 large tomato, coarsely chopped

Using a paring knife, make cross-hatch cuts in the flesh of each avocado half, cutting down to the skin but not through it. Use a spoon to scoop the flesh from the skins and place it in a medium bowl. Mash roughly with a fork. Stir in the onion, chili, coriander, salt and lime juice, then fold in the tomato. Transfer the guacamole to a bowl and serve right away, or squeeze additional lime juice on top to prevent oxidation, then cover and refrigerate for up to 4 hours.

Any leftover guacamole can be stored in an airtight container in the fridge for up to 2 days, but add a little more lime juice and the avocado stone to prevent oxidation.

Nutritional analysis per serving (115 g): *Calories: 202, Fat: 21 g, Saturated Fat: 3 g, Cholesterol: 110 mg, Fiber: 8 g, Protein: 3 g, Carbohydrates: 16 g, Sodium: 900 mg*

ALMOND HUMMUS

Here's a chickpea-free twist on hummus, made with raw almonds that have been soaked to render them more digestible. Use it as a dip, spread or side dish, or in any way you'd use traditional hummus.

Makes: 750 g
Prep time: 15 minutes, plus soaking time

- 85 g raw almonds
- 145 g sesame seeds
- 30 g fresh parsley leaves
- 2 teaspoons ground cumin
- 2 garlic cloves
- juice of 2 lemons
- 1 tablespoon sea salt
- 4 tablespoons extra-virgin olive oil

Put the almonds in a bowl and cover with 1 litre filtered water. Set aside to soak for 8 to 12 hours at room temperature (depending how much time you have).

Drain the almonds and rinse well.

Combine the almonds, sesame seeds, parsley, cumin, garlic, lemon juice and salt in a food processor and pulse until roughly ground, 5 or 6 pulses. Scrape down the sides of the bowl. With the machine running, add the olive oil and 60 ml filtered water in a steady stream and process until the mixture is creamy, about 1 minute.

Transfer the hummus to a bowl and serve right away, or refrigerate in an airtight container for up to 4 days. Serve with chicory leaves, cucumber sticks or other cut veggies.

Nutritional analysis per serving (185 g): *Calories: 338, Fat: 23 g, Saturated Fat: 2 g, Cholesterol: 0 mg, Fiber: 5 g, Protein: 11 g, Carbohydrates: 26 g, Sodium: 684 mg*

ROMESCO HUMMUS

PEGAN DIET

Chickpeas, the main ingredient in hummus, are fibrous nutritional beans. Beans can cause blood sugar to spike, so I don't recommend this dip during the *Eat Fat, Get Thin* 21–day plan, but if you find that beans agree with you, you'll love this hummus with a flavorful twist.

Makes: about 750 g
Prep time: 10 minutes

- 2 x 400-g cans chickpeas, rinsed and drained
- 2 tablespoons fresh lemon juice
- 125 ml Pecan Romesco (page 270)
- 125 ml extra-virgin olive oil
- 2 teaspoons sea salt
- ¼ teaspoon freshly ground black pepper

Pulse the chickpeas in a food processor until coarsely but uniformly ground, 5 or 6 pulses. Scrape down the sides of the bowl, add the lemon juice and Pecan Romesco sauce, and process until combined, about 30 seconds. With the machine running, add the olive oil in a slow, steady stream. Scrape down the bowl, add the salt and pepper, and process until well combined, about 1 minute.

Transfer to a bowl and serve right away, or refrigerate in an airtight container for up to 4 days.

Nutritional analysis per serving (185 g): *Calories: 259, Fat: 21 g, Saturated Fat: 2 g, Cholesterol: 0 mg, Fiber: 6 g, Protein: 6 g, Carbohydrates: 19 g, Sodium: 916 mg*

ARTICHOKE DIP WITH CRUDITÉS

Artichoke dip is a family favorite that I make whenever we have guests over. Artichokes are under-utilized, impressively nutritious veggies, but some people are put off by the time-consuming prep they need. Don't be! Simply purchase them in cans—they are just as good for you—you'll find that they quickly become regular items on your shopping list. In this dip, I use nutritional yeast, my favorite replacement for inflammatory cheese.

Makes: about 900 g
Prep time: 15 minutes

- 1 x 400-g can artichoke hearts, rinsed, drained and roughly chopped
- 450 g Homemade Mayonnaise (page 265)
- 75 g fresh parsley leaves, roughly chopped
- leaves from 1 large thyme sprig, finely chopped
- 2 tablespoons fresh lemon juice
- 2 tablespoons nutritional yeast
- 1 teaspoon sea salt
- 3 celery sticks, cut into 5-cm sticks
- 1 large carrot, scrubbed and cut into batons
- 1 small daikon radish, peeled and cut into 5-mm rounds

Put the artichokes in a large bowl, add the mayonnaise, parsley, thyme, lemon juice, nutritional yeast and salt and stir together. Transfer the mixture to a serving bowl and serve with the celery and carrot sticks and the daikon rounds.

Any leftover dip can be stored in an airtight container in the fridge for up to 4 days.

Nutritional analysis per serving (115 g): *Calories: 123, Fat: 0 g, Saturated Fat: 0 g, Cholesterol: 0 mg, Fiber: 3 g, Protein: 2 g, Carbohydrates: 6 g, Sodium: 440 mg*

"Cheesy" Sunflower Seed Dip

In this recipe, vitamin E-rich sunflower seed butter (which resembles peanut butter) is transformed into a dip that's perfect with cucumber and pepper sticks, and any other vegetables in your fridge. For a flavor change, try adding a few tablespoons of fresh chopped herbs, such as parsley, dill and coriander.

Makes: about 450 g
Prep time: 5 minutes

- 225 g sunflower seed butter
- 4 tablespoons extra-virgin olive oil
- 4 tablespoons apple cider vinegar
- 2 tablespoons wheat-free tamari
- 3 tablespoons nutritional yeast
- 2 garlic cloves

Combine all the ingredients in a blender and add 2 tablespoons filtered water. Blend on high speed until smooth and creamy, about 1 minute.

Transfer the dip to a bowl and serve right away, or refrigerate in an airtight container for up to 4 days.

Nutritional analysis per serving (115 g): *Calories: 272, Fat: 24 g, Saturated Fat: 2 g, Cholesterol: 0 mg, Fiber: 2 g, Protein: 7 g, Carbohydrates: 9 g, Sodium: 190 mg*

CREAMY HORSERADISH DIP

This simple dip works really well with vegetable crudités, or as a sauce for grilled steaks or rich, oily fish, such as salmon and trout.

Makes: about 250 g
Prep time: 5 minutes

- 220 g Homemade Mayonnaise (page 265)
- 2 tablespoons horseradish sauce, or to taste (its heat can vary enormously)
- 1 tablespoon apple cider vinegar
- sea salt

Put the mayonnaise, horseradish and vinegar in a small bowl and stir together. Season to taste with salt. Serve right away with crudités, or refrigerate in an airtight container for up to 1 week.

Nutritional analysis per serving (60 g): *Calories: 99, Fat: 11 g, Saturated Fat: 1.75 g, Cholesterol: 5.5 mg, Fiber: 0 g, Protein: 0 g, Carbohydrates: 0.25 g, Sodium: 100 mg*

TAHINI SPREAD WITH-GARLIC-SHALLOT OIL AND PARSLEY

Tahini, a paste made from sesame seeds, is a staple in my pantry. I like to use it as a base for dressings and sauces. Here I use it in a spread that's perfect with crudités and crackers.

Makes: 450 g
Prep time: 15 minutes
Cook time: 5 minutes

- 125 ml extra-virgin olive oil
- 1 large shallot, thinly sliced into rounds
- 3 garlic cloves, crushed
- leaves from 2 large thyme sprigs, finely chopped
- 345 g tahini
- 30 g parsley leaves, roughly chopped
- 2 tablespoons apple cider vinegar
- 2 teaspoons sea salt

Warm the olive oil, shallot and garlic in a medium frying pan over a low heat until the oil is infused with flavor, 5 to 6 minutes. Remove from the heat, stir in the thyme and allow to cool completely.

Put the tahini in a medium bowl, add the parsley, vinegar, salt and oil mixture and stir together. Serve right away, or refrigerate in an airtight container for up to 1 week.

Nutritional analysis per serving (115 g): *Calories: 262, Fat: 25 g, Saturated Fat: 3 g, Cholesterol: 0 mg, Fiber: 3 g, Protein: 5 g, Carbohydrates: 7 g, Sodium: 410 mg*

ROASTED PARSNIP AND ALMOND SPREAD WITH SUN-DRIED TOMATOES

Parsnip is an earthy, naturally sweet and fiber-rich root vegetable that is particularly delicious when roasted. Serve this creamy spread as a snack or appetizer with roasted or raw vegetables, or as an accompaniment to roasted or grilled meats.

Makes: about 500 g
Prep time: 10 minutes
Cook time: 30 minutes

- 450 g parsnips, peeled and trimmed
- 45 g unsalted roasted almonds
- 2 garlic cloves
- 6 sun-dried tomatoes in olive oil
- grated zest of 1 lemon
- 1 teaspoon dried thyme
- 1 teaspoon dried oregano
- 2 teaspoons sea salt
- ¼ teaspoon freshly ground black pepper

Preheat the oven to 160°C/325°F/Gas 3.

Place the parsnips in a 33 x 23-cm baking dish and pour in 250 ml filtered water. Cover with foil and bake until the parsnips are tender, 25 to 30 minutes. Remove from the oven, transfer the parsnips to a cutting board, and allow to cool completely. Cut each parsnip into 4 to 6 pieces.

Put the almonds and garlic in a food processor and process until well ground, about 45 seconds. Scrape down the sides of the bowl, then add the parsnips, sun-dried tomatoes, lemon zest, thyme, oregano, salt and pepper. Process until the mixture is well puréed, about 1 minute.

Transfer the spread to a bowl and serve right away, or refrigerate in an airtight container for up to 4 days.

Nutritional analysis per serving (115 g): *Calories: 330, Fat: 20 g, Saturated Fat: 2 g, Cholesterol: 0 mg, Fiber: 11 g, Protein: 10 g, Carbohydrates: 33 g, Sodium: 901 mg*

WALNUT AND CARAMELIZED ONION PÂTÉ

Enjoy this delicious spread with roasted veggies or on crackers.

Makes: about 300 g
Prep time: 15 minutes
Cook time: 15 minutes

- 200g raw walnuts
- 1½ tablespoons Ghee (page 279)
- 1 large onion, thinly sliced
- 3 garlic cloves
- leaves from 4 thyme sprigs, finely chopped
- 2 teaspoons sea salt
- ¼ teaspoon freshly ground black pepper
- 1 tablespoon apple cider vinegar
- 3 tablespoons extra-virgin olive oil

Preheat the oven to 180°C/350°F/Gas 4. Spread the walnuts on a baking sheet and toast in the oven until golden brown, 8 to 10 minutes.

Meanwhile, in a medium frying pan, warm the ghee over a medium-high heat until melted. Add the onion and cook, stirring occasionally, until softened and golden brown, 10 to 12 minutes. Transfer to a plate and allow to cool to room temperature.

Put the toasted walnuts in a food processor, add the garlic, thyme, salt and pepper and pulse until the walnuts are roughly chopped, 6 to 7 pulses. Add the caramelized onion and vinegar and process until smooth, about 45 seconds. With the machine running, add the olive oil in a slow, steady stream and process until fully incorporated.

Transfer the pâté to a 1-litre glass jar or dish. Serve right away, or cover and refrigerate for up to 5 days.

Nutritional analysis per serving (75 g): *Calories: 535, Fat: 54 g, Saturated Fat: 8 g, Cholesterol: 13 mg, Fiber: 5 g, Protein: 10 g, Carbohydrates: 12 g, Sodium: 887 mg*

Devilled Eggs

After years of being vilified, eggs are now recognized as a great source of high-quality fat and protein. This is an easy-to-prepare, crowd-pleasing appetizer.

Makes: 24
Prep time: 15 minutes
Cook time: 15 minutes

- 12 large eggs
- 30 g parsley leaves
- 50 g Homemade Mayonnaise (page 265)
- 1 tablespoon apple cider vinegar
- 2 teaspoons Dijon mustard
- 1½ teaspoons sea salt
- 1 teaspoon garlic powder
- ¼ teaspoon chipotle chili powder

Place the eggs in a large saucepan and add enough filtered water to cover by about 2.5 cm. Bring to the boil over a high heat and cook for 1 minute. Immediately remove the pan from the heat, cover and set aside for 5 minutes. Meanwhile, fill a large bowl with iced water.

Pour off the water in the pan, then carefully transfer the eggs to the iced water. Set aside until completely cooled, then remove the eggs.

Carefully crack and peel the eggs, then cut each in half lengthways. Pop the yolks into a food processor and arrange the whites in a single layer in a baking dish or on a serving platter. Add the parsley to the food processor and pulse until combined, about 3 pulses. Add the mayonnaise, vinegar, mustard, salt, garlic powder and chipotle powder and process until thoroughly mixed, about 30 seconds.

Pipe or spoon the yolk mixture equally into the egg whites. Serve right away, or refrigerate in an airtight container for up to 3 days.

Nutritional analysis per serving (4 halves): *Calories: 221, Fat: 15 g, Saturated Fat: 3 g, Cholesterol: 353 mg, Fiber: 1 g, Protein: 13 g, Carbohydrates: 4 g, Sodium: 320 mg*

DIY Nori Bites

This is a fun buffet-style snack and a great appetizer for a casual get–together.

Serves: 4
Prep time: 10 minutes, plus soaking time

- 90 g pumpkin seeds
- 2 garlic cloves
- 2 celery sticks, cut into 2.5-cm pieces
- 35 g drained kimchi or sauerkraut
- 4 tablespoons extra-virgin olive oil
- ½ teaspoon sea salt
- 4 tablespoons fresh lemon juice
- 8 nori sheets, cut into quarters
- 200 g sprouts (such as sunflower, buckwheat or radish)
- 2 avocados, stoned, peeled and sliced 5 mm thick
- hot sauce, for serving (optional)

Put the pumpkin seeds in a bowl and cover with 1 litre filtered water. Set aside to soak for 2 to 3 hours at room temperature. Drain and rinse well.

Put the drained seeds in a food processor, add the garlic, celery and kimchi and pulse until combined, then process until crumbly, about 45 seconds. Scrape down the bowl, add the olive oil, salt and lemon juice and process until combined. With the machine running, slowly add up to 125 ml filtered water in a steady stream until the mixture is spreadable, with the consistency of thick nut butter. Transfer to a serving bowl.

To serve, set out the pumpkin seed mixture and the nori, sprouts, avocado and hot sauce, if using. Get your guests to make their own nori bites, as follows: spread pumpkin seed mixture on a piece of nori, top with sprouts and avocado, and sprinkle with hot sauce, if desired.

Nutritional analysis per serving (8 pieces): *Calories: 593, Fat: 49 g, Saturated Fat: 4 g, Cholesterol: 0 mg, Fiber: 30 g, Protein: 20 g, Carbohydrates: 22.6 g, Sodium: 340 mg*

CRISPY TEMPEH TRIANGLES

Tempeh is a fermented soya bean product rich in protein, so it's a great alternative to meat. Fermentation makes the soya easier to digest and also increases its nutrition. These triangles are a yummy snack to pack in a lunch to take to work or school.

Serves: 4
Prep time: 5 minutes
Cook time: 10 minutes

- 1 x 225-g block organic, GMO-free tempeh
- 4 tablespoons coconut oil
- 1 teaspoon sea salt

Cut the tempeh in half horizontally, then cut each half on the diagonal into quarters. You will have a total of 8 triangles.

Warm the coconut oil in a large frying pan over a medium–high heat until shimmering. Add the tempeh triangles in a single layer, sprinkle with ½ teaspoon of the salt, and cook until browned and crisp, 3 to 4 minutes. Carefully flip each triangle, sprinkle with the remaining salt, and cook until the underside too is browned and crisp, about 2 minutes.

Transfer the tempeh to a plate lined with kitchen paper. Allow to cool for a minute or so, then serve.

Nutritional analysis per serving (2 triangles): *Calories: 227, Fat: 20 g, Saturated Fat: 13 g, Cholesterol: 0 mg, Fiber: 0 g, Protein: 11 g, Carbohydrates: 5 g, Sodium: 565 mg*

CHOPPED SARDINES ON CUCUMBER SLICES

Gram for gram, sardines are one of the best sources of the omega−3 fatty acids EPA and DHA, both of which have been shown to lower triglycerides and total cholesterol levels. This simple, flavorful snack offers great nourishment whenever you need a little energy boost. Be sure to look for sardines packed in olive oil.

Serves: 4
Prep time: 5 minutes

- 1 small cucumber, sliced into 5-mm rounds
- 1 x 120-g can sardines packed in olive oil
- juice of ½ lemon
- 1 tablespoon fresh dill, roughly chopped
- 1 small shallot, finely chopped
- ¼ teaspoon cayenne pepper

Arrange the cucumber slices on a plate.

Pour 2 tablespoons of the oil from the sardines into a small bowl. Roughly chop the sardines, then add them to the bowl with the oil. Add the lemon juice (discarding any pips), the dill, shallot and cayenne. Stir until combined.

Spoon the sardine mixture onto the cucumber slices, spreading it evenly, and serve.

Nutritional analysis per serving: *Calories: 58, Fat: 3 g, Saturated Fat: 1 g, Cholesterol: 17 mg, Fiber: 4 g, Protein: 4 g, Carbohydrates: 9 g, Sodium: 45 mg*

Roasted Bone Marrow

Delicious, deeply nourishing bone marrow is a great source of omega−3 fatty acids, vitamins and minerals. Roasted marrow can be spread on gluten-free crackers, stirred into soups, or folded into scrambled eggs. Or you can enjoy spoonfuls of the rich, buttery texture and flavor on its own.

Serves: 4
Prep time: 2 minutes
Cook time: 15 minutes

- 900 g beef marrowbones

Preheat the oven to 230°C/450°F/Gas 8.

Place the marrowbones in a roasting pan. Roast until the bones are golden brown and the marrow is soft, about 15 minutes.

Scoop the marrow out of the bones and serve.

Nutritional analysis per serving (30 g): *Calories: 299, Fat: 20 g, Saturated Fat: 9 g, Cholesterol: 0 mg, Fiber: 0 g, Protein: 25 g, Carbohydrates: 2 g, Sodium: 315 mg*

8

Salads

FARMERS' MARKET SALAD WITH MISO DRESSING

There's nothing I love more than a salad made with ingredients fresh from the local farmers' market.

Serves: 4
Prep time: 20 minutes

- 125 ml extra-virgin olive oil
- 2 tablespoons soya-free miso
- 2 tablespoons red wine vinegar
- 2 tablespoons fresh lemon juice
- 1 large courgette, trimmed
- 1 large yellow summer squash, trimmed
- 350 g mixed salad leaves
- 1 large cucumber, thinly sliced into rounds
- 4 radishes, very thinly sliced
- 12 cherry tomatoes, cut in half
- 1 avocado, stoned, peeled and cut into chunks
- 4 tablespoons toasted shelled sunflower seeds

Put the olive oil in a bowl, add the miso, vinegar and lemon juice and whisk together. Set this dressing aside.

Using a spiralizer or a vegetable peeler, cut the courgette and summer squash into spaghetti–size spirals.

Divide the salad leaves equally between 4 serving bowls. Top with the courgette and squash spirals, followed by the cucumber, radishes, tomatoes and avocado chunks, evenly dividing the ingredients.

Whisk the dressing to recombine, then drizzle it over the salad. Sprinkle each serving with 1 tablespoon of the sunflower seeds and serve.

Nutritional analysis per serving: *Calories: 442, Fat: 35 g, Saturated Fat: 5 g, Cholesterol: 0 mg, Fiber: 7 g, Protein: 6 g, Carbohydrates: 20 g, Sodium: 381 mg*

Rocket, Cucumber and Avocado Salad with Raspberry-Coriander Vinaigrette

This salad is simple, light and refreshing, perfect at the height of summer when raspberries are in season. At other times of the year, the vinaigrette can be made with frozen raspberries that have been defrosted: the salad will still be beautiful *and* delicious.

Serves: 4
Prep time: 20 minutes

- 350g baby rocket
- 1 large cucumber, peeled and thinly sliced into rounds
- 2 avocados, stoned, peeled and cut into small chunks
- 125 g raspberries
- 125 ml extra-virgin olive oil
- 4 tablespoons apple cider vinegar
- 1 teaspoon ground coriander
- 1 teaspoon sea salt
- ¼ teaspoon freshly ground black pepper
- leaves from 2 mint sprigs, thinly sliced

Spread out the rocket on a large platter and top with the cucumber slices and avocado chunks.

Combine the raspberries, olive oil, vinegar, coriander, salt and pepper in a blender and blend on high speed until smooth, about 30 seconds. Strain the vinaigrette through a fine-mesh sieve set over a bowl, using a flexible spatula to push the purée through; discard the seeds in the sieve.

Drizzle the vinaigrette over the salad, sprinkle with the mint and serve.

Nutritional analysis per serving: *Calories: 410, Fat: 38 g, Saturated Fat: 5 g, Cholesterol: 0 mg, Fiber: 8 g, Protein: 3 g, Carbohydrates: 18 g, Sodium: 665 mg*

ENDIVE AND GRAPEFRUIT SALAD WITH SHERRY VINAIGRETTE

PEGAN DIET

Endive, which resembles frilly lettuce, has a slightly bitter flavor. Bitter foods naturally detoxify the liver and stimulate enzyme production in the digestive system. Bitter notes also help to balance out sweet, sour and salty flavors.

Serves: 4
Prep time: 15 minutes, plus time to tenderize

- 2 grapefruits
- 4 tablespoons extra-virgin olive oil
- 2 tablespoons sherry vinegar
- 1 tablespoon Dijon mustard
- 1 small shallot, finely chopped
- ½ teaspoon sea salt
- 1 large head endive, core removed, leaves very thinly sliced
- 60 g toasted walnuts, coarsely chopped

Cut the top and bottom off a grapefruit. Stand it on a chopping board and, using a sharp knife, cut away the rind and white pith in strips from top to bottom. Slide the blade down each side of the membrane dividing the segments to separate the flesh. Repeat with the remaining grapefruit.

Put the olive oil in a small bowl, add the vinegar, mustard, shallot and salt and whisk together.

Place the endive in a large bowl, drizzle the dressing over it and toss gently until evenly coated. Allow them to sit for 10 minutes to tenderize.

Divide the endive between 4 plates, sprinkle with the walnuts, and top with the grapefruit segments. Serve.

Nutritional analysis per serving: *Calories: 300, Fat: 24 g, Saturated Fat: 7 g, Cholesterol: 0 mg, Fiber: 4 g, Protein: 5 g, Carbohydrates: 22 g, Sodium: 330 mg*

Shaved Asparagus and Radicchio Salad

Most people are familiar with roasted or steamed asparagus, but this springtime vegetable can also be enjoyed raw. The trick is to shave the stalks into thin, noodle-like strips so that they're tender and pleasing to eat. A sharp Y-shaped vegetable peeler is the best tool for the job.

Serves: 4
Prep time: 20 minutes

- 1 bunch thick-stalked asparagus, trimmed
- 1 head radicchio, cored and thinly sliced
- 35 g pine nuts, toasted
- 3 tablespoons extra-virgin olive oil
- 2 tablespoons fresh lemon juice
- ½ teaspoon sea salt
- ¼ teaspoon freshly ground black pepper

Lay the asparagus on a cutting board and use a Y-shaped vegetable peeler to shave the spears from top to bottom, creating long, thin slices.

Place the strips in a large bowl, add the remaining ingredients and toss gently to combine.

Divide the salad between 4 plates and serve.

Nutritional analysis per serving: *Calories: 177, Fat: 16 g, Saturated Fat: 2 g, Cholesterol: 0 mg, Fiber: 3 g, Protein: 5 g, Carbohydrates: 7 g, Sodium: 282 mg*

Super Green Salad

Massaging olive oil and salt into kale gently wilts the leaves so that they taste lightly cooked. When you don't feel like doing much cooking on a hot summer day, this is a perfect, ultra-healthy, super-quick dish to prepare.

Serves: 4
Prep time: 20 minutes

- 2 bunches curly kale, stemmed and torn into small pieces
- 3 tablespoons extra-virgin olive oil
- 1 teaspoon sea salt
- 1 orange (any kind, optional for Pegan Diet)
- 200 g shredded red cabbage
- 225 g broccoli, stems removed, florets cut into-bite-sized pieces
- 2 avocados, stoned, peeled and cut into large chunks
- 3 tablespoons spirulina
- 2 tablespoons hemp seeds
- 2 tablespoons fresh lemon juice
- 1 teaspoon dried thyme
- 1 teaspoon dried oregano

Put the kale, olive oil and salt. Use your hands to gently massage the leaves, helping them to soften and wilt. Set aside to stand for 5 minutes.

Meanwhile, cut the top and bottom off the orange, if using. Stand it on a chopping board and, using a sharp knife, cut away the rind and white pith in strips from top to bottom. Slide the blade down each side of the membrane dividing the segments to separate the flesh.

Add the orange sections and all the remaining ingredients to the kale. Toss to combine, then serve.

Nutritional analysis per serving: *Calories: 540, Fat: 37 g, Saturated Fat: 5 g, Cholesterol: 0 mg, Fiber: 25 g, Protein: 17 g, Carbohydrates: 44 g, Sodium: 728 mg*

HEARTY SPINACH SALAD

Here's a satisfying salad full of healthy fats from olives, olive oil, eggs and avocado. If you want to boost the protein content, add slices of grilled chicken, steak or tofu.

Serves: 4
Prep time: 10 minutes
Cook time: 15 minutes

- 4 large eggs
- 12 green beans, trimmed
- 1 tablespoon extra-virgin olive oil
- 30 g baby spinach
- 1 avocado, stoned, peeled and cut into chunks
- 1 small red onion, thinly sliced
- 200g pitted Kalamata olives
- about 125 ml Rosemary Vinaigrette (page 273)

Place the eggs in a saucepan and add enough filtered water to cover by 2.5 cm. Bring to the boil and cook for 1 minute. Immediately cover and set aside for 5 minutes. Meanwhile, fill a large bowl with iced water.

Drain the eggs and transfer them to the iced water. When completely cold, wipe the eggs dry (reserving the ice bath for later). Crack and peel the eggs, then cut them in half lengthways. Set aside.

Fill a saucepan with 1 litre filtered water and bring to a simmer over a medium–high heat. Add the green beans and cook until al dente, about 3 minutes. Drain immediately and transfer the beans to the iced water to stop them cooking. Once chilled, drain again and transfer to a small bowl. Drizzle with the olive oil and toss to combine.

Divide the spinach between 4 plates and place 2 egg halves on each portion. Top equally with the beans, avocado, onion and olives. Drizzle each salad with 2 tablespoons of vinaigrette and serve.

Nutritional analysis per serving: *Calories: 238, Fat: 18 g, Saturated Fat: 3 g, Cholesterol: 175 mg, Fiber: 6 g, Protein: 9 g, Carbohydrates: 13 g, Sodium: 578 mg*

Avocado, Celery and Citrus Salad

PEGAN DIET

I love the combination of ingredients in this hydrating salad, which features a variety of textures, good-quality fats and a bright citrus blast. It's great at any time of year when you're craving refreshment. If you want to add a little protein to make this a complete meal, incorporate some thinly sliced grilled chicken breast.

Serves: 4
Prep time: 15 minutes

- 3 tablespoons Homemade Mayonnaise (page 265)
- 1 tablespoon fresh lemon juice
- 1 tablespoon poppy seeds
- ½ teaspoon sea salt
- 2 blood oranges or Valencia oranges
- 1 small head romaine lettuce, torn into bite-sized pieces
- 2 avocados, stoned, peeled and each half cut into 4 slices
- 4 celery sticks, thinly sliced

To make the dressing, put the mayonnaise in a small bowl with the lemon juice, poppy seeds and salt and whisk together. If desired, add 1 to 2 tablespoons filtered water to thin the dressing.

Cut the top and bottom off an orange. Stand it on a chopping board and, using a sharp knife, cut away the rind and white pith in strips from top to bottom, following the contour of the fruit. Cut the flesh into thin rounds. Repeat with the remaining orange.

Divide the lettuce between 4 plates, then top equally with the orange rounds, avocado slices and celery. Drizzle some dressing over each salad and serve.

Nutritional analysis per serving: *Calories: 309, Fat: 20 g, Saturated Fat: 2 g, Cholesterol: 5 mg, Fiber: 11 g, Protein: 5 g, Carbohydrates: 31 g, Sodium: 603 mg*

ARTICHOKE, AVOCADO AND CUCUMBER SALAD

You don't always need lettuce to make a salad. The simple, fresh flavors in this quick-to-prepare dish are a great addition to any lunch or dinner. The salad is also great as a topping for grain-free breads or crackers.

Serves: 4
Prep time: 10 minutes, plus marinating time

- 4 tablespoons extra-virgin olive oil
- 2 tablespoons red wine vinegar
- 1 garlic clove, crushed
- 2 teaspoons fresh dill, roughly chopped
- ½ teaspoon sea salt
- ¼ teaspoon freshly ground black pepper
- 2 large cucumbers, trimmed
- 1 x 400-g can artichoke hearts, rinsed, drained and roughly chopped
- 1 large avocado, stoned, peeled and cut into chunks

To make the dressing, put the olive oil, vinegar, garlic, dill, salt and pepper in a small bowl and whisk together.

Slice the cucumbers lengthways into quarters, then cut each quarter widthways into 1-cm chunks.

Combine the cucumbers, artichoke hearts and avocado chunks in a large bowl. Whisk the dressing to recombine, then pour it over the salad and toss well. Set aside for 10 minutes to allow the flavors to mingle. Serve.

Nutritional analysis per serving: *Calories: 528, Fat: 30 g, Saturated Fat: 3 g, Cholesterol: 0 mg, Fiber: 10 g, Protein: 13 g, Carbohydrates: 61 g, Sodium: 958 mg*

HEARTS OF PALM CHOPPED SALAD

This fantastic recipe with Mexican flair requires very little effort to prepare, and absolutely no cooking, but the result is a flavorful, hearty salad. Enhance the dish with some grilled chicken or wild salmon and you will be satisfied for hours.

Serves: 4
Prep time: 20 minutes

- 4 tablespoons extra-virgin olive oil
- 2 tablespoons fresh lime juice
- 2 teaspoons fresh oregano leaves, finely chopped
- 1 teaspoon sea salt
- ¼ teaspoon freshly ground black pepper
- ¼ teaspoon dried red chili flakes
- 2 large avocados, stoned, peeled and cut into-bite-sized chunks
- 1 x 400-g can hearts of palm, rinsed, drained and sliced into rounds 5 mm thick
- 1 large sweet red pepper, seeded and chopped
- 190 g cherry tomatoes, cut in half
- ½ small red onion, finely diced
- 3 tablespoons toasted unsalted pumpkin seeds
- 2 tablespoons chopped fresh coriander leaves

To make the dressing, combine the olive oil, lime juice, oregano, salt, black pepper and red pepper flakes in a screwtop jar and shake well. The dressing can be refrigerated for up to 2 weeks; bring to room temperature before using.

Put the avocado in a large bowl and add the hearts of palm, red pepper, cherry tomatoes and red onion. Shake the vinaigrette to recombine, drizzle it over the salad, and toss gently to mix. Sprinkle the salad with the pumpkin seeds and coriander and serve.

Nutritional analysis per serving: *Calories: 297, Fat: 27 g, Saturated Fat: 4 g, Cholesterol: 0 mg, Fiber: 6 g, Protein: 5 g, Carbohydrates: 15 g, Sodium: 804 mg*

CAULIFLOWER-HEMP SEED "TABBOULEH"

Cauliflower is a fantastic low-carb vegetable that can be transformed to mimic rice and other grains. In this recipe, it replaces the bulgur wheat that's used in traditional tabbouleh.

Serves: 4
Prep time: 30 minutes, plus chiling time

- 1 head cauliflower, trimmed
- 40 g hemp seeds
- 1 bunch parsley, stemmed and roughly chopped
- 2 large tomatoes, cored and diced
- 1 cucumber, diced
- 1 large shallot, finely chopped
- 3 garlic cloves, crushed
- 4 tablespoons extra-virgin olive oil
- grated zest and juice of 1 lemon
- 1 teaspoon sea salt

Using a chef's knife, cut the head of cauliflower in half, then use a paring knife to cut the florets away from the core. Cut the florets into roughly 2.5-cm pieces.

Put about half the florets in a food processor and pulse until broken into fine bits that resemble grains of rice, 4 or 5 one-second pulses. Transfer to a large bowl and repeat with the remaining cauliflower.

Add all the remaining ingredients to the cauliflower and toss well to combine. Cover and refrigerate for at least 2 hours, or up to 3 days. Toss to recombine and serve chilled or at room temperature.

Nutritional analysis per serving: *Calories: 271, Fat: 19 g, Saturated Fat: 2 g, Cholesterol: 0 mg, Fiber: 9 g, Protein: 10 g, Carbohydrates: 24 g, Sodium: 648 mg*

Wild Rice and Cavolo Nero Salad

PEGAN DIET

This super-satisfying salad is a terrific accompaniment.

Serves: 4
Prep time: 20 minutes, plus soaking time
Cook time: 25 minutes, plus cooling time

- 160 g wild rice
- 2 bunches cavolo nero, stemmed and torn into 2.5-cm pieces
- 4 tablespoons extra-virgin olive oil
- 1 teaspoon sea salt
- ¼ teaspoon freshly ground black pepper
- 6 large Brussels sprouts, trimmed and shredded
- 1 large carrot, scrubbed and shredded
- ½ red onion, finely chopped
- 2 tablespoons fresh lemon juice
- 10 g toasted pumpkin seeds

Put the wild rice in a bowl, cover with 1 litre filtered water and leave to soak overnight at room temperature. Drain and rinse well.

Place the rice in a small saucepan and add 625 ml filtered water. Cover, bring to the boil over a high heat, then simmer until the rice is tender and has absorbed all the liquid, about 20 minutes. Spread out the rice in a shallow baking dish and allow to cool to room temperature.

Place the cavolo nero in a large bowl, drizzle with the olive oil, then sprinkle with the salt and pepper. Using your fingers, gently massage the leaves until wilted.

Add the wild rice plus all the remaining ingredients and toss. Serve.

Nutritional analysis per serving: *Calories: 294, Fat: 19 g, Saturated Fat: 3 g, Cholesterol: 0 mg, Fiber: 7 g, Protein: 11 g, Carbohydrates: 26 g, Sodium 633 mg*

Quinoa and Black Bean Salad with Mexican Flavors

PEGAN DIET

In the last ten years, quinoa has gone from a virtually unknown grain (actually a seed) to a beloved superfood. Naturally gluten-free and loaded with protein, it's a healthy and hearty addition to your diet. This Mexican-inspired salad is great served with grilled chicken or fish.

Serves: 4
Prep time: 20 minutes
Cook time: 20 minutes, plus cooling time

- 170 g quinoa, rinsed and drained
- 1 x 400-g can black beans, rinsed and drained
- 2 avocados, stoned, peeled and cut into small chunks
- 1 large sweet red pepper, seeded and finely diced
- 1 large tomato, finely diced
- ½ bunch coriander, roughly chopped
- 4 tablespoons extra-virgin olive oil
- 2 tablespoons fresh lime juice
- 2 teaspoons ground cumin
- generous pinch of chipotle powder
- 1 teaspoon sea salt, plus more as needed

Place the quinoa in a saucepan and cover with 500 ml filtered water. Bring to the boil over a high heat, then cover and simmer until the quinoa is almost tender and has absorbed all the liquid, about 15 minutes. Set aside, covered, for 5 minutes. Using a fork, fluff the quinoa, then spread it out in a shallow baking dish and allow to cool to room temperature.

Transfer the cooled quinoa to a large bowl and add all the remaining ingredients. Toss until well combined, then taste and adjust the seasoning with more salt, if needed. Serve.

Nutritional analysis per serving: *Calories: 466, Fat: 24 g, Saturated Fat: 3 g, Cholesterol: 0 mg, Fiber: 9 g, Protein: 12 g, Carbohydrates: 54 g, Sodium: 969 mg*

Mediterranean Sardine Salad

Small oily fish are among the most nutrient-dense foods you can eat. They are also one of the more sustainable seafood options. Canned sardines play a central role in this simple but delicious salad. For a creamier version, replace the olive oil with an equal amount of Homemade Mayonnaise (page 265).

Serves: 4
Prep time: 15 minutes

- 4 x 120-g cans sardines in water or olive oil, drained
- 2 celery sticks, finely chopped
- 1 small shallot, finely chopped
- 2 garlic cloves, crushed
- 6 sun-dried tomatoes in olive oil, finely chopped
- leaves from 2 large basil sprigs, thinly sliced
- 2 tablespoons apple cider vinegar
- 4 tablespoons extra-virgin olive oil
- ½ teaspoon sea salt
- ½ teaspoon freshly ground black pepper
- 300 g baby salad greens

Place the sardines in a bowl and mash them with a fork. Add the celery, shallot, garlic, sun-dried tomatoes and basil and stir to incorporate. Add the vinegar, olive oil, salt and pepper and stir until well combined.

Divide the greens between 4 plates. Top each with a portion of the sardine mixture and serve.

Nutritional analysis per serving: Calories: 353, Fat: 28 g, Saturated Fat: 4 g, Cholesterol: 100 mg, Fiber: 1 g, Protein: 18 g, Carbohydrates: 9 g, Sodium: 568 mg

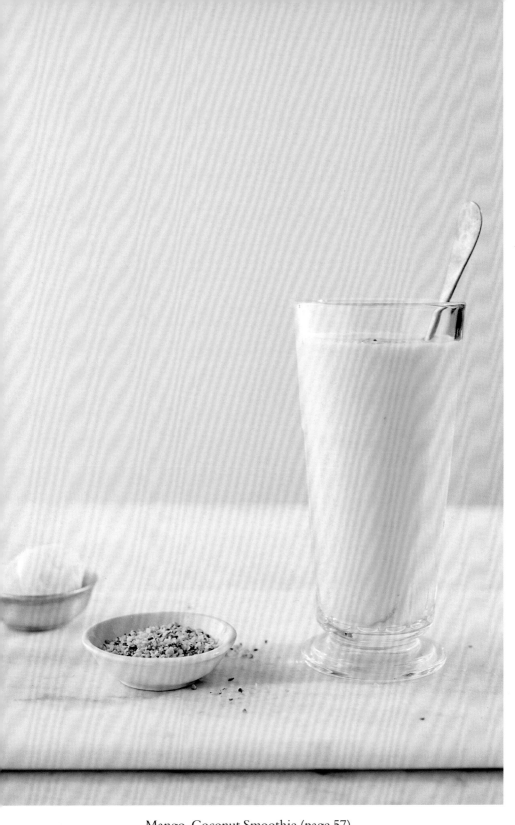

Mango–Coconut Smoothie (page 57)

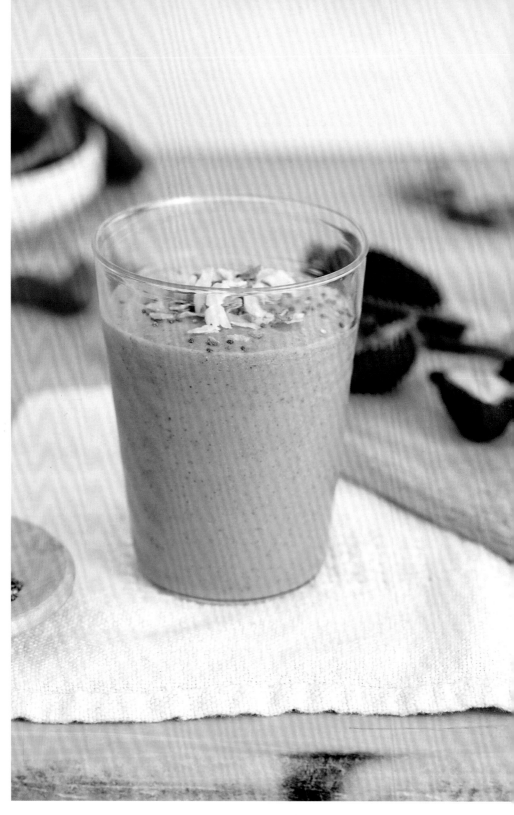

Omega-3 Green Smoothie (page 62)

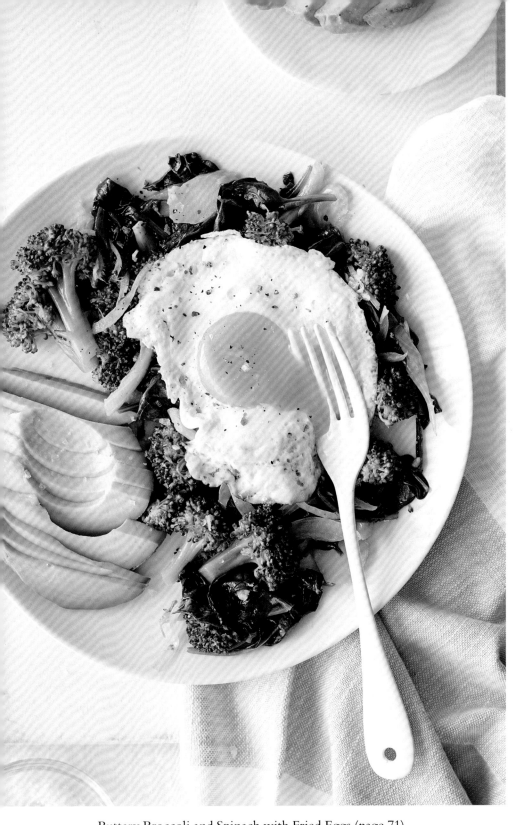

Buttery Broccoli and Spinach with Fried Eggs (page 71)

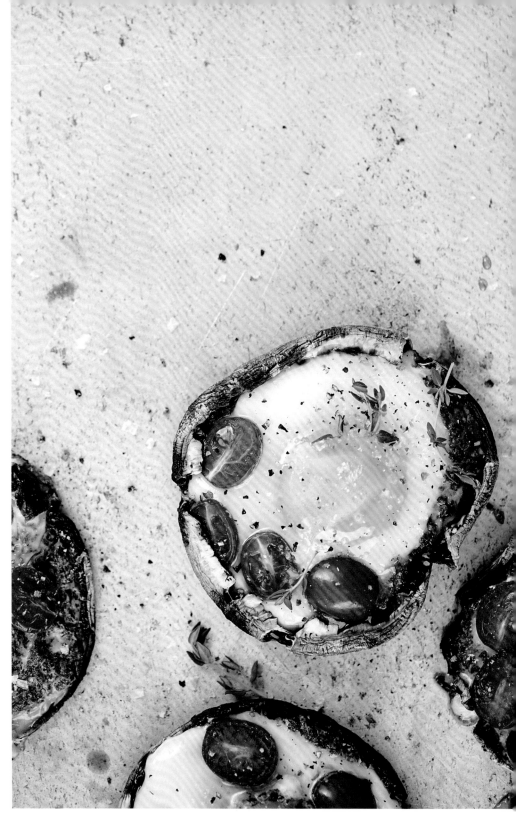

Eggs Baked on Portobello Mushrooms (page 74)

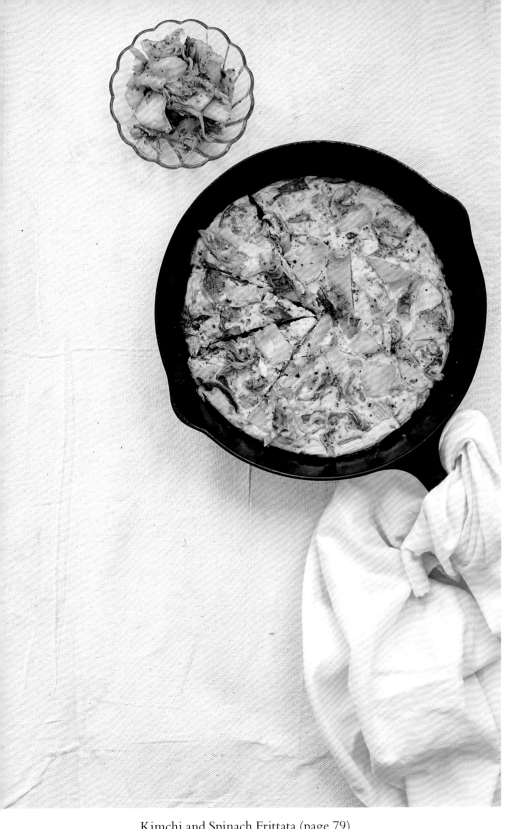

Kimchi and Spinach Frittata (page 79)

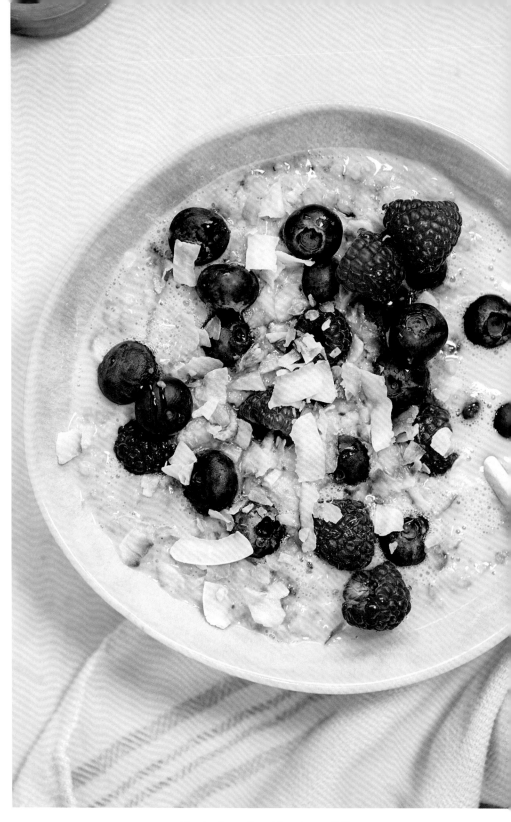

Buckwheat Porridge (page 84)

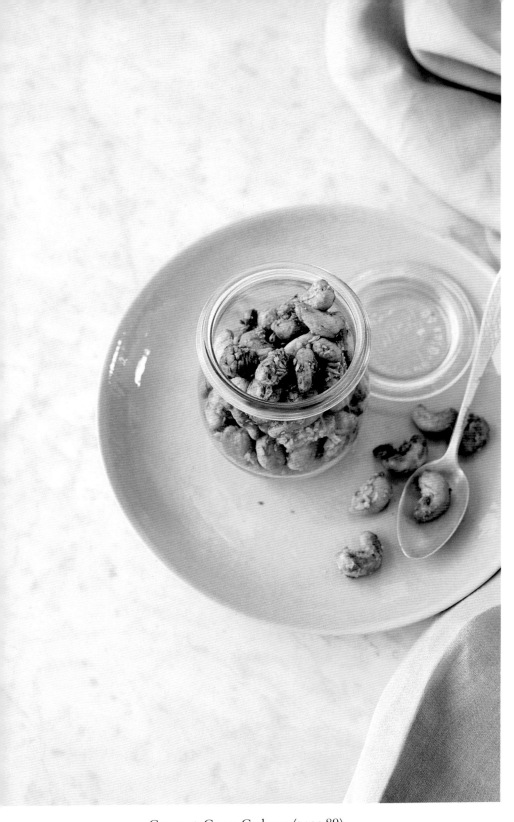

Coconut-Curry Cashews (page 89)

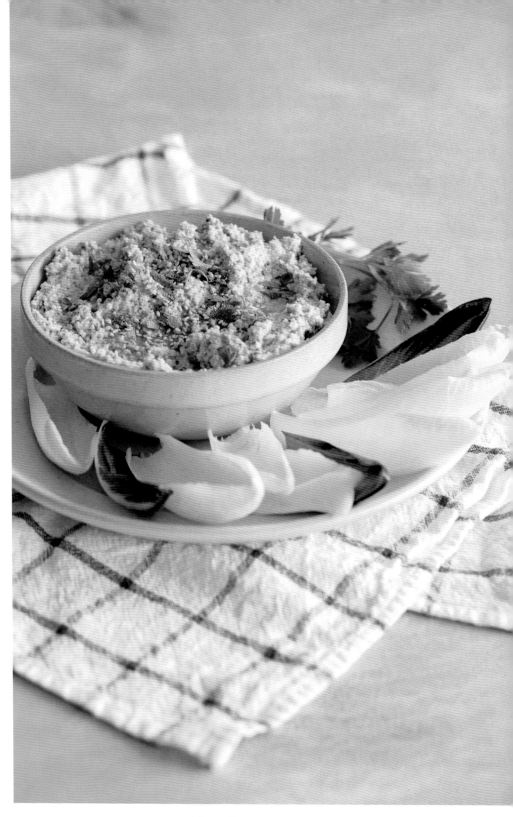

Almond Hummus (page 94)

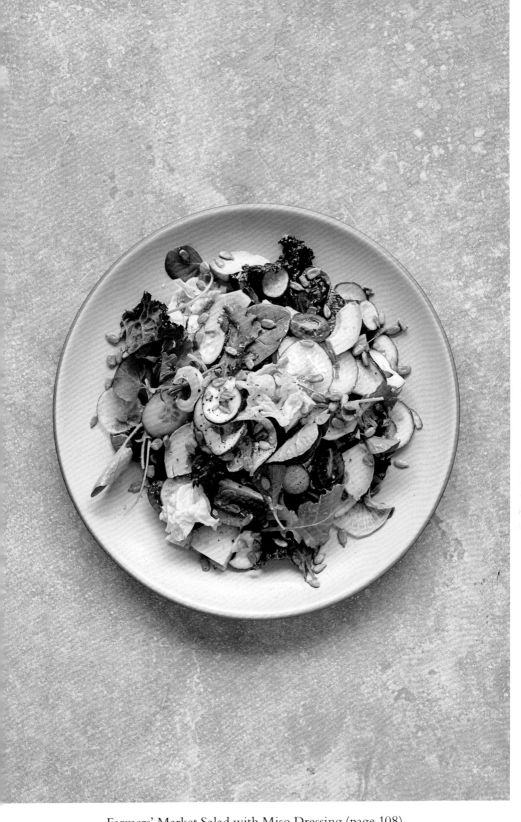

Farmers' Market Salad with Miso Dressing (page 108)

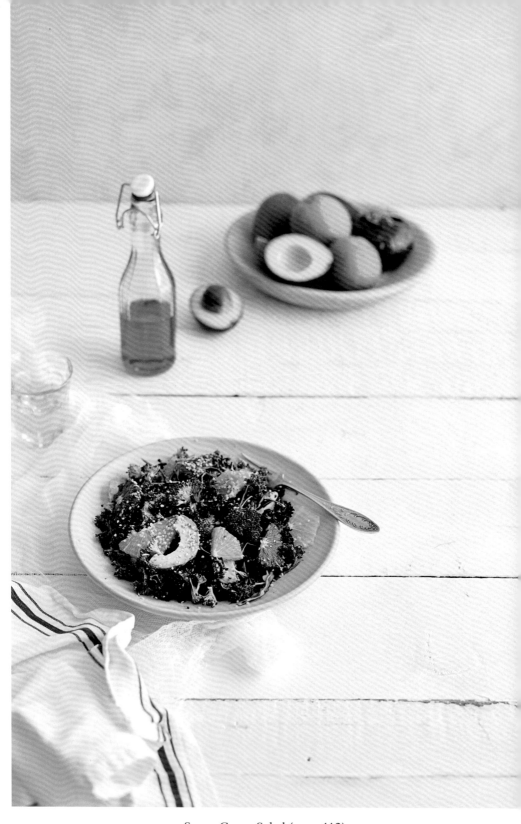

Super Green Salad (page 112)

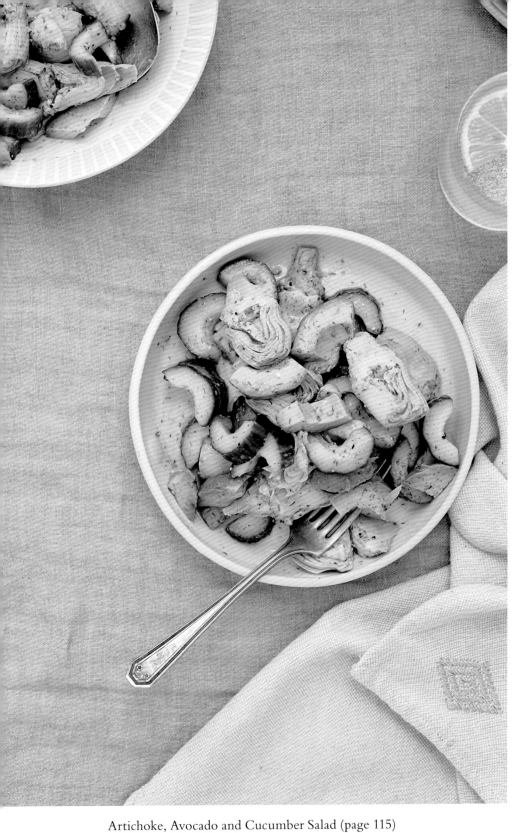

Artichoke, Avocado and Cucumber Salad (page 115)

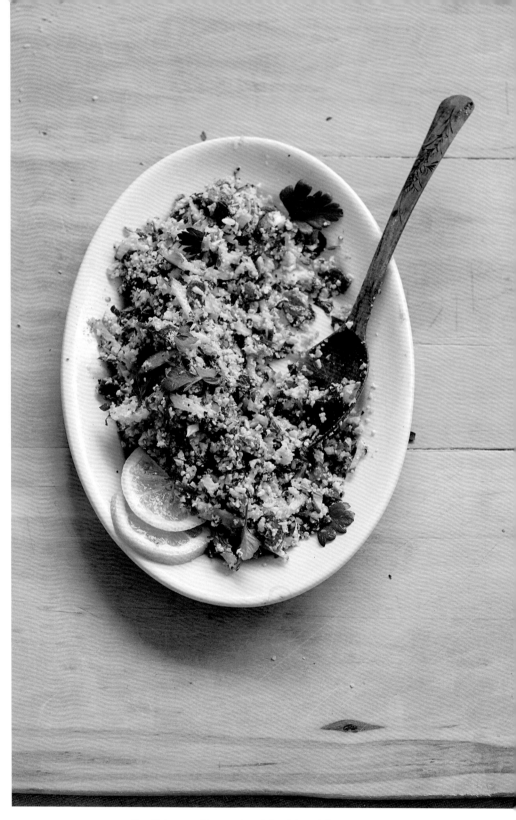

Cauliflower–Hemp Seed "Tabbouleh" (page 117)

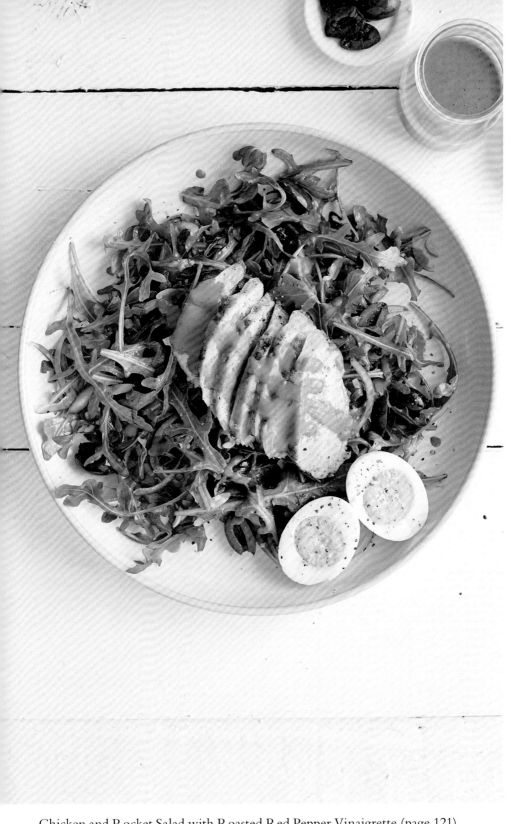

Chicken and Rocket Salad with Roasted Red Pepper Vinaigrette (page 121)

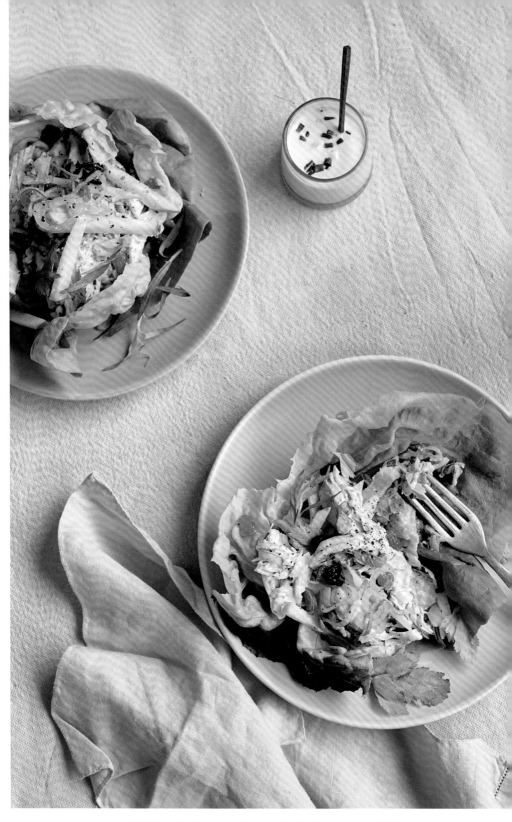

Waldorf Salad with Roasted Chicken (page 123)

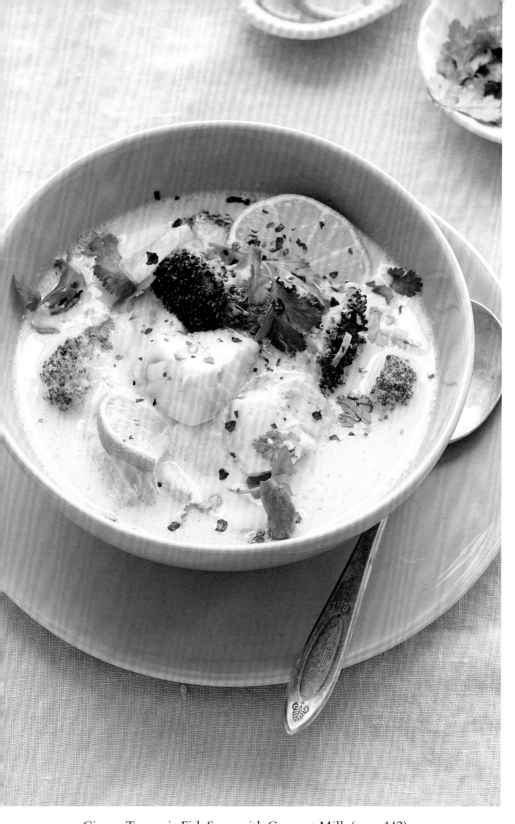

Ginger–Turmeric Fish Soup with Coconut Milk (page 142)

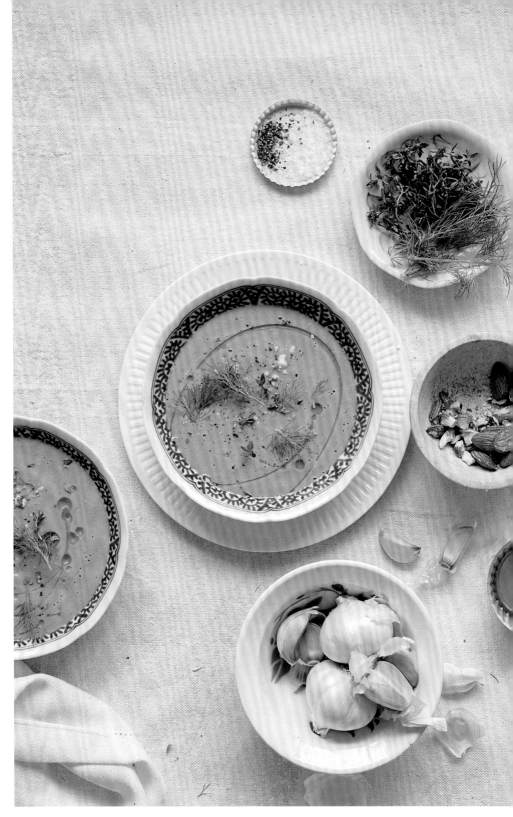

Creamy Fennel and Mushroom Soup (page 146)

CHICKEN AND ROCKET SALAD WITH ROASTED RED PEPPER VINAIGRETTE

This is a great main-course salad that combines high-quality fats from eggs, olives and extra-virgin olive oil. If you have chicken left over from another meal, use it in place of the chicken breasts and the dish will come together in just a few minutes.

Serves: 4
Prep time: 15 minutes
Cook time: 10 minutes

- 4 x 175-g boneless, skinless chicken breasts
- ¼ teaspoon freshly ground black pepper
- 1 teaspoon sea salt
- 2 tablespoons avocado oil
- 2 roasted red peppers from a jar, patted dry
- 4 tablespoons extra-virgin olive oil
- 2 tablespoons sherry vinegar
- 2 garlic cloves
- ½ teaspoon dried thyme
- 40 g baby rocket
- 1 small red onion, thinly sliced
- 200 g pitted Kalamata olives
- 2 hard-boiled eggs, peeled and quartered

Preheat the oven to 180°C/350°F/Gas 4.

Season the chicken breasts on both sides with the pepper and ½ teaspoon of the salt.

Warm the avocado oil in a large ovenproof frying pan over a medium-high heat until shimmering. Add the chicken breasts to the pan in a single layer and cook for 5 minutes. Flip the breasts, transfer the pan to the oven, and cook until the meat is opaque throughout and the internal temperature reaches 75°C/165°F on an instant-read thermometer, about 6 to 7 minutes. Transfer the chicken breasts to a cutting board and leave to rest for 2 to 3 minutes while you make the vinaigrette.

Combine the roasted red peppers, olive oil, vinegar, garlic, thyme and the remaining ½ teaspoon salt in a blender. Blend on high speed until smooth, about 30 seconds.

Cut the chicken breasts widthways into 1-cm slices. Divide the rocket between 4 plates and top with the onion slices, olives, hard-boiled eggs and chicken, evenly distributing the ingredients. Drizzle some of the vinaigrette over each salad and serve.

Nutritional analysis per serving: Calories: 507, Fat: 30 g, Saturated Fat: 4 g, Cholesterol: 171 mg, Fiber: 2 g, Protein: 32 g, Carbohydrates: 8 g, Sodium: 1122 mg

WALDORF SALAD WITH ROASTED CHICKEN

PEGAN DIET

This classic salad was created at the Waldorf Hotel in New York in the late 1800s and traditionally combines apples, walnuts, celery and raisins in a creamy dressing. The version below includes roasted chicken for protein, and the Homemade Mayo in the dressing adds healthy fats.

Serves: 4
Prep time: 10 minutes
Cook time: 15 minutes

- 2 x 175-g boneless, skin-on chicken breasts
- ¼ teaspoon freshly ground black pepper
- 2 tablespoons extra-virgin olive oil
- 165 g Homemade Mayonnaise (page 265)
- 2 tablespoons apple cider vinegar
- 1 tablespoon Dijon mustard
- 1 tablespoon finely chopped fresh chives
- 1 small shallot, thinly sliced
- 1 Granny Smith apple, cored and cut into 1-cm chunks
- 75 g raw walnuts, roughly chopped
- 3 celery sticks, sliced 5 mm thick
- 35 g raisins
- 1 butterhead lettuce, leaves separated

Preheat the oven to 180°C/350°F/Gas 4.

Place the chicken breasts in a small baking dish, season on both sides with the pepper, and drizzle with the olive oil. Turn the breasts skin-side down and roast until the meat is opaque throughout and the internal temperature reaches 75°C/165°F on an-instant-read thermometer, 12 to 15 minutes. Transfer the breasts to a cutting board and allow to cool.

Meanwhile, put the mayonnaise, vinegar, mustard, chives and shallot into a small bowl and whisk together.

Cut the cooled chicken into 1-cm chunks and place in a large bowl. Add the apple, walnuts, celery, raisins and the dressing and fold until the mixture is well combined.

Arrange the lettuce leaves on 4 plates, dividing them equally. Scoop the salad mixture onto the lettuce and serve.

Nutritional analysis per serving: Calories: 576, Fat: 38 g, Saturated Fat: 5 g, Cholesterol: 45 mg, Fiber: 0 g, Protein: 14 g, Carbohydrates: 61 g, Sodium: 139 mg

Taco Salad

While this salad contains all the spicy flavors of minced beef tacos, it isn't weighed down by the heaviness of corn, a common allergen. It's a meal the whole family will love.

Serves: 4
Prep time: 30 minutes
Cook time: 10 minutes

- 1 tablespoon coconut oil
- 450 g grass-fed minced beef
- 2 teaspoons ground cumin
- 1 teaspoon ground coriander
- ¼ teaspoon chipotle powder
- 1 teaspoon dried oregano
- 1 teaspoon sea salt
- 1 avocado, stoned, peeled and cut into large chunks
- 2 tablespoons extra-virgin olive oil
- 4 g fresh coriander leaves
- 1 garlic clove
- juice of 1 lime
- ¼ teaspoon cayenne pepper
- 70–80 g mesclun (mixed salad green, e.g. lamb's lettuce, rocket, chicory)
- 200 g shredded red cabbage
- 2 carrots, scrubbed and shredded
- 1 large tomato, cut into large chunks

Warm the coconut oil in a large frying pan over a medium–high heat until shimmering. Add the beef and cook for 2 minutes, stirring frequently and breaking it into pieces with a wooden spoon. Add the cumin, dried coriander, chipotle powder, oregano and ½ teaspoon of the salt and continue to cook, stirring occasionally, until the beef is cooked through, about 4 minutes.

Meanwhile, put the avocado, olive oil, fresh coriander, garlic, lime juice, cayenne and the remaining ½ teaspoon salt in a blender, add 65 ml filtered water and blend on high speed until smooth, about 45 seconds. Transfer the dressing to a small serving bowl.

Put the mesclun in a large bowl with the cabbage, carrots and tomato and toss to combine. Divide equally between 4 plates and top with the beef mixture. Serve with the dressing offered separately.

Nutritional analysis per serving: Calories: 500, Fat: 31 g, Saturated Fat: 11 g, Cholesterol: 70 mg, Fiber: 17 g, Protein: 28 g, Carbohydrates: 37 g, Sodium: 713 mg

9

Broths and Soups

Dr. Hyman's Veggie-Bone Broth

Believe the hype! Bone broth is one of the most healing foods you can sip. It's good for your hair, skin, nails, digestion, immune system and gut.

Makes: 1.75 to 2 litres
Prep time: 10 minutes
Cook time: 15 to 27 hours (unattended), plus cooling time

- 1.75 kg bones, preferably organic
- 2 tablespoons apple cider vinegar
- 2 carrots, scrubbed and roughly chopped
- 2 celery sticks, roughly chopped
- 1 onion, chopped
- 2 garlic cloves, crushed
- 2 bay leaves
- 1 bunch parsley
- 1 tablespoon sea salt

Place the bones in a 4-litre slow cooker or stockpot and drizzle the vinegar over them. Add the remaining ingredients and pour in 2 litres filtered water. Stir to combine. If using a slow cooker: cover, set it to low, and cook for 12 to 24 hours. If using a stockpot: place it over a high heat and bring to the boil, then lower the heat to medium and simmer for 8 to 12 hours (depending on how much time you have).

Using a slotted spoon, remove and discard the bones, vegetables and herbs. Pour the liquid through a fine sieve into a large glass container and allow to cool. Cover and refrigerate until cold, at least 3 hours.

Using a spoon, skim off and discard the layer of solidified fat on the surface. Refrigerate in an airtight container for up to 4 days, or freeze for up to 1 year.

Nutritional analysis per serving (500 ml): *Calories: 34, Fat: 0 g, Saturated Fat: 0 g, Cholesterol: 0 mg, Fiber: 2 g, Protein: 2 g, Carbohydrates: 8 g, Sodium: 918 mg*

MISO-BUTTER BROTH

Miso is a Japanese fermented paste traditionally made with soya beans, but there are many soya-free miso options out there, so shop around. Miso-spiked soup boosts the immune system, so sip this broth when you feel sluggish or have a cold coming on.

Serves: 1
Prep time: 5 minutes

- 375 ml hot Veggie-Bone Broth (page 128)
- 1 tablespoon soya-free miso
- 1½ tablespoons unsalted, grass-fed butter

Place all the ingredients in a blender and blend on a high speed until well combined, about 30 seconds. Pour the broth into a mug and drink immediately.

Nutritional analysis per serving: *Calories: 193, Fat: 17 g, Saturated Fat: 10 g, Cholesterol: 43 mg, Fiber: 0 g, Protein: 1 g, Carbohydrates: 8 g, Sodium: 1514 mg*

Mineral-Rich Green Soup

In the heat of summer, simple raw soups like this are exactly what I crave. The miso in this recipe not only adds delicious flavor, it also delivers an array of beneficial bacteria that aid in digestion and help nurture a healthy gut.

Serves: 4
Prep time: 10 minutes

- 2 avocados, stoned, peeled and quartered
- 2 large tomatoes, cored and cut into chunks
- 2 large handfuls baby spinach
- 2 garlic cloves
- 3 spring onions, roughly chopped
- 2 tablespoons fresh mint leaves
- 2 tablespoons fresh coriander leaves
- juice of 1 lemon
- 2 tablespoons soya-free miso
- 4 tablespoons extra-virgin olive oil
- ¼ teaspoon freshly ground black pepper
- 375 ml chilled herbal tea (e.g. holy basil, nettle or lemon balm)

Place all the ingredients in a blender with 275 ml of the herbal tea. Blend on a high speed until smooth and creamy, about 30 seconds. Blend in the remaining tea as needed to thin the soup to the desired consistency. Serve right away or refrigerate in an airtight container for up to 1 day.

Nutritional analysis per serving: *Calories: 487, Fat: 24 g, Saturated Fat: 3 g, Cholesterol: 0 mg, Fiber: 5 g, Protein: 3 g, Carbohydrates: 91 g, Sodium: 262 mg*

CURRIED COURGETTE-AVOCADO SOUP

Courgette is typically paired with Mediterranean flavors, but with a touch of curry powder for spice and avocado for richness, this recipe livens things up a bit. At the height of summer, when the weather is warm, this soup can be enjoyed chilled.

Serves: 4
Prep time: 10 minutes
Cook time: 10 minutes

- 2 tablespoons Ghee (page 279)
- 2 large courgette, cut into thin rounds
- 1 large shallot, sliced into thin rounds
- sea salt
- 2 avocados, stoned and peeled; 1 diced for garnish
- 2 tablespoons fresh lime juice
- 2 teaspoons curry powder
- 4 tablespoons extra-virgin olive oil
- ½ small bunch coriander, stemmed and roughly chopped

Warm the ghee in a saucepan over a medium heat until melted. Add the courgette and shallot, sprinkle with a little salt, and cook, stirring occasionally, until softened and translucent, 5 to 6 minutes.

Transfer the courgette mixture to a blender. Add the flesh from 1 avocado along with the lime juice, curry powder and olive oil. Blend on a high speed until smooth and creamy, about 45 seconds. If the soup is too thick, add up to 65 ml filtered water to thin it. Season to taste with salt.

Divide the soup between 4 bowls. Garnish with the coriander and diced avocado and serve.

Nutritional analysis per serving: *Calories: 336, Fat: 32 g, Saturated Fat: 8 g, Cholesterol: 0 mg, Fiber: 7 g, Protein: 4 g, Carbohydrates: 13 g, Sodium: 584 mg*

Chunky Vegetable and Adzuki Bean Soup with Miso

PEGAN DIET

Savory miso is known for its ability to boost the immune system. Kombu is a wild-harvested seaweed that imparts an earthy flavor and has properties to help cook the beans quicker and make them more digestible.

Serves: 4
Prep time: 30 minutes, plus soaking time
Cook time: 1½ hours

- 200 g dried adzuki beans
- 1 small piece kombu
- 1 large leek, white section halved lengthways, rinsed and cut into chunks
- 225 g cremini mushrooms, quartered
- 2 large carrots, scrubbed and cut into rounds 5 mm thick
- 1 large turnip, peeled and cut into 1-cm chunks
- 2.5-cm piece fresh ginger, peeled and finely chopped
- 40 g dried wakame (broken into small pieces if in long strands)
- 1 bunch cavolo nero, stemmed and cut into small pieces
- 65 ml soya-free miso

Put the adzuki beans and kombu in a bowl and cover with 1.5 litres filtered water. Leave to soak overnight at room temperature. Drain well.

Put the beans and kombu in a very large saucepan with the leek, mushrooms, carrots, turnip, ginger and wakame. Pour in 1 litre filtered water and bring to a simmer over a medium-high heat. Reduce the heat to medium and cook, stirring occasionally, until the beans are tender, about 1 hour; add more water as needed.

Stir in the cavolo nero and cook until tender, about 15 minutes.

Spoon 1 tablespoon of the miso into each of 4 serving bowls. Ladle about 375 ml of the soup into each bowl and serve.

Nutritional analysis per serving (375 ml): *Calories: 355, Fat: 3 g, Saturated Fat: 0 g, Cholesterol: 0 mg, Fiber: 16 g, Protein: 20 g, Carbohydrates: 66 g, Sodium: 1305 mg*

SUMMER BOUNTY VEGETABLE STEW

PEGAN DIET

Summer vegetables at their peak of freshness, taste and nutrition are the high-light of this hearty stew. Cumin, chili powder, coriander and lime juice lend the dish bold Mexican flavor accents.

Serves: 4
Prep time: 20 minutes
Cook time: 45 minutes

- 2 tablespoons Ghee (page 279)
- 1 large onion, thinly sliced
- 2 celery sticks, sliced 5 mm thick
- 1 large carrot, scrubbed and cut into rounds 5 mm thick
- 2 garlic cloves, crushed
- 2 large tomatoes, cored and roughly chopped
- 1 sweet red pepper, seeded and thinly sliced
- 2 teaspoons ground cumin
- 1 teaspoon chili powder
- 1 teaspoon dried oregano
- 1 litre Dr. Hyman's Veggie-Bone Broth (page 128)
- 1 courgette, sliced into rounds 1 cm thick
- 200 g green beans, trimmed and cut into thirds
- 1 x 400-g can chickpeas, rinsed and drained
- 4 g fresh coriander leaves, roughly chopped
- juice of 1 lime

Warm the ghee in a large saucepan over a medium heat until melted. Add the onion, celery and carrots and cook, stirring occasionally, until slightly softened, 3 to 4 minutes. Stir in the garlic, tomatoes, red pepper, cumin, chili powder and oregano, then pour in the bone broth. Bring to the boil, then simmer until the vegetables are tender, about 15 minutes.

Add the courgette, green beans and chickpeas and stir to combine. Continue to simmer until slightly thickened and the courgette and beans are tender, 15 to 20 minutes. Stir in the coriander and lime juice. Serve.

Nutritional analysis per serving: Calories: 374, Fat: 11 g, Saturated Fat: 5 g, Cholesterol: 15 mg, Fiber: 30 g, Protein: 16 g, Carbohydrates: 59 g, Sodium: 518 mg

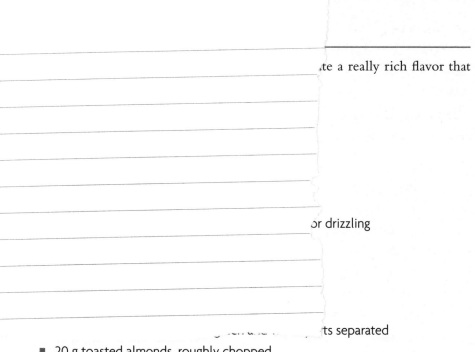

.te a really rich flavor that

or drizzling

ts separated

- 20 g toasted almonds, roughly chopped

Preheat the oven to 190°C/375°F/Gas 5.

Chop the cauliflower in half, then cut the florets into roughly 1-cm pieces.

Place the cauliflower in a bowl with the onion, olive oil, salt and pepper. Toss until the vegetables are evenly coated, then spread in an even layer on a baking sheet. Roast until the cauliflower is golden brown, stirring occasionally, about 20 minutes.

Transfer the cauliflower mixture to a large saucepan and add the almond milk, bay leaf and white parts of the spring onions. Bring to the boil over a medium–high heat, then reduce the heat and simmer until the vegetables are completely tender, about 20 minutes.

Discard the bay leaf. Using a stick blender, purée the mixture until mostly smooth but still with some chunks. Season to taste.

Ladle the soup into bowls. Sprinkle with the almonds and the green parts of the spring onions, drizzle with extra olive oil, and serve.

Nutritional analysis per serving: *Calories: 226, Fat: 16 g, Saturated Fat: 2 g, Cholesterol: 0 mg, Fiber: 7 g, Protein: 5 g, Carbohydrates: 17 g, Sodium: 224 mg*

Sweet Potato Soup with Coconut and Ginger

I love silky, smooth soups like this one.

Serves: 4
Prep time: 15 minutes
Cook time: 30 minutes

- 2 tablespoons Ghee (page 279)
- 1 large onion, thinly sliced
- 4 garlic cloves, crushed
- 2.5-cm piece fresh ginger, peeled and finely chopped
- 900 g sweet potatoes, peeled and cut into 5-mm rounds
- 1 litre Dr. Hyman's Veggie-Bone Broth (page 128)
- 125 ml full-fat coconut milk
- 1 teaspoon sea salt
- 4 spring onions, thinly sliced
- 4 tablespoons unsalted, grass-fed butter

Warm the ghee in a 4-litre saucepan over a medium heat until melted. Add the onion and cook, stirring occasionally, until softened and translucent, 3 to 4 minutes. Stir in the garlic and ginger and cook until fragrant, about 2 minutes. Add the sweet potatoes, stir to incorporate, then pour in the bone broth. Bring the liquid to a simmer, cover and cook until the sweet potatoes are tender, about 20 minutes.

Pour a batch of soup and some of the coconut milk into a blender, ensuring it is no more than half full, as hot liquids need room for expansion. Cover the lid with a folded tea towel and hold it down as you blend, gradually increasing to high speed. Return the mixture to a clean saucepan, then blend the rest of the soup and coconut milk in the same way.

Warm the blended soup over a medium heat, then stir in the salt and spring onions. Ladle the soup into 4 bowls. Top each portion with 1 tablespoon of the butter and serve.

Nutritional analysis per serving: *Calories: 520, Fat: 23 g, Saturated Fat: 14 g, Cholesterol: 35 mg, Fiber: 8 g, Protein: 9 g, Carbohydrates: 58 g, Sodium: 744 mg*

CREAMY POTATO SOUP WITH DULSE FLAKES

PEGAN DIET

Dulse is a wild seaweed loaded with vitamins and minerals, including B_6, B_{12}, iron and potassium. It has a unique flavor that adds a delicious, savory character to this creamy soup. You can find dried dulse flakes in most healthfood stores.

Serves: 4
Prep time: 15 minutes
Cook time: 45 minutes

- 2 tablespoons Ghee (page 279)
- 1 large onion, thinly sliced
- 3 celery sticks, sliced 5 mm thick
- 3 garlic cloves, crushed
- 1.25 kg Yukon Gold potatoes or other non-waxy variety, peeled and cut into quarters
- 1 litre chicken or vegetable stock
- 1 tablespoon dried thyme
- 1 teaspoon ground fennel seeds
- 1 bay leaf
- 4 tablespoons unsalted, grass-fed butter
- 2 tablespoons dulse flakes
- ½ teaspoon freshly ground white pepper

Warm the ghee in a large saucepan over a medium–high heat until melted. Add the onion and celery and cook, stirring occasionally, until the vege-tables are slightly softened, 3 to 4 minutes. Stir in the garlic and cook until fragrant, about 1 minute. Add the potatoes, stock, thyme, fennel seeds and bay leaf. Bring to the boil, then reduce the heat and simmer uncovered, stirring occasionally, until the potatoes are very tender, about 30 minutes.

Remove and discard the bay leaf. Place about half the soup mixture in a blender along with 2 tablespoons of the butter and blend on high speed until creamy. Do not fill the blender more than halfway, as hot liquids expand when blending. Also, cover the lid with a folded tea towel and hold it down as you blend, starting slowly and gradually increasing to high speed. Transfer to a bowl and repeat this process with the remaining soup mixture and butter.

Return the puréed soup to the saucepan and warm over a medium heat, stirring occasionally, until hot. Stir in the dulse flakes and white pepper and serve.

Nutritional analysis per serving: *Calories: 402, Fat: 12 g, Saturated Fat: 6 g, Cholesterol: 11 mg, Fiber: 6 g, Protein: 13 g, Carbohydrates: 63 g, Sodium: 410 mg*

Rich Onion Soup

Onions contain powerful phytochemicals that can help reduce inflammation.

Serves: 4
Prep time: 15 minutes
Cook time: 1 hour

- 1 tablespoon Ghee (page 279)
- 1.25 kg onions, thinly sliced
- 250 ml dry white wine
- 2 bay leaves
- 3 garlic cloves, crushed
- 1 piece kombu, 5 x 15 cm
- 1 tablespoon dried thyme
- 2 teaspoons dried oregano
- 2 litres Dr. Hyman's Veggie-Bone Broth (page 128)
- 2 tablespoons wheat-free tamari
- 6 tablespoons unsalted grass-fed butter, at room temperature
- ½ bunch parsley, stemmed and roughly chopped

Warm the ghee in a large saucepan over a medium–high heat until melted. Add the onions and cook, stirring occasionally, until softened and golden brown, 15 to 20 minutes. Pour in the wine and add the bay leaves, garlic, kombu, thyme and oregano. Simmer until the wine has reduced by half, then pour in the bone broth. Bring to a simmer, then cook at a gentle simmer, partially covered, for 45 minutes.

Stir the tamari into the soup. Remove and discard the bay leaves and kombu and ladle the soup into 4 serving bowls. Top each portion with 1½ tablespoons of the butter, sprinkle with parsley and serve.

Nutritional analysis per serving: *Calories: 621, Fat: 27 g, Saturated Fat: 14 g, Cholesterol: 56 mg, Fiber: 24 g, Protein: 28 g, Carbohydrates: 66 g, Sodium: 755 mg*

Hearty Lentil and Mushroom Soup

PEGAN DIET

Here is a classic lentil soup with a twist: cremini mushrooms make the protein-rich soup even heartier and give it a deep, meaty flavor. Leftovers keep well, so make a double batch and enjoy the soup over the course of a week.

Serves: 4
Prep time: 20 minutes, plus soaking time
Cook time: 1¾ hours

- 300 g green lentils
- 2 tablespoons Ghee (page 279)
- 1 large onion, roughly chopped
- 300 g thinly sliced cremini mushrooms
- 3 celery sticks, cut into 1-cm pieces
- 2 large carrots, scrubbed and cut into 5-mm rounds
- 1 litre Dr. Hyman's Veggie-Bone Broth (page 128) or filtered water
- 30 g dulse flakes
- 2 bay leaves
- 2 teaspoons garlic powder
- leaves from a 15-cm rosemary sprig, finely chopped
- 1 teaspoon dried basil
- ½ teaspoon freshly ground black pepper, or to taste
- ½ bunch parsley, stemmed and roughly chopped

Put the lentils in a bowl and cover with 1 litre filtered water. Leave to soak overnight at room temperature.

Drain the lentils in a colander and set aside.

Warm the ghee in a 4-litre saucepan over a medium–high heat until melted. Add the onion and mushrooms and cook, stirring occasionally, until softened, 3 to 4 minutes. Stir in the celery, carrots and lentils and cook until heated through. Add the bone broth, dulse flakes, bay leaves, garlic powder, rosemary and basil and stir to combine. Cover and bring to the boil, then reduce the heat and simmer until the lentils and vegetables are completely tender, about 1½ hours.

Season the soup with the pepper. Stir in the parsley and serve.

Nutritional analysis per serving: *Calories: 234, Fat: 8 g, Saturated Fat: 5 g, Cholesterol: 2 mg, Fiber: 11 g, Protein: 12 g, Carbohydrates: 30 g, Sodium: 2968 mg*

Ginger-Turmeric Fish Soup with Coconut Milk

Ginger and turmeric are ingredients with anti-inflammatory properties, and both infuse this soup with exotic fragrance and flavor. For the best taste and texture, I recommend using at least two different kinds of white fish, but the soup will still be delicious if made with only one.

Serves: 4
Prep time: 20 minutes
Cook time: 30 minutes

- 1 tablespoon Ghee (page 279)
- 1 small onion, thinly sliced
- 1 tablespoon peeled and finely chopped ginger
- 1 tablespoon peeled and finely chopped fresh turmeric or 1 teaspoon ground turmeric
- 2 garlic cloves, crushed
- 1 x 400-ml can-full-fat coconut milk
- 500 ml chicken stock
- 2 tablespoons fish sauce
- 1 tablespoon rice vinegar
- 1 large head broccoli, stems peeled and finely diced, florets cut into 2.5-cm pieces
- 450 g skinless white fish fillets (such as cod, halibut, haddock or seabass), cut into 2.5-cm chunks
- 8 g fresh coriander leaves, roughly chopped
- dried red chili flakes, to garnish (optional)
- 1 lime, cut into 8 wedges

Warm the ghee in a large flameproof casserole dish over amedium heat until melted. Add the onion and cook, stirring occasionally, until softened and translucent, 3 to 4 minutes. Stir in the ginger, turmeric and garlic and cook until fragrant, about 1 minute. Add the coconut milk, chicken stock, fish sauce and vinegar, bring to a simmer, and cook for 10 minutes. Stir in the broccoli and cook until tender, about 5 minutes. Add the fish, stir gently and cook until it is opaque throughout, about 5 minutes. Gently stir in the coriander.

Ladle the soup into bowls, garnish with the chili flakes, if using, and serve with the lime wedges on the side.

Nutritional analysis per serving: *Calories: 314, Fat: 15 g, Saturated Fat: 10 g, Cholesterol: 54 mg, Fiber: 4 g, Protein: 27 g, Carbohydrates: 19 g, Sodium: 1016 mg*

Chicken, Vegetable and Lentil Soup

PEGAN DIET

This is comfort food at its best. Nutritious veggies combined with healing bone broth, protein-dense lentils and chicken yield a soup that's a complete lunch or dinner in a bowl.

Serves: 4
Prep time: 30 minutes
Cook time: 1 hour

- 2 tablespoons coconut oil
- 1 large onion, thinly sliced
- 2 celery sticks, sliced 5 mm thick
- 2 small carrots, scrubbed and cut into 5-mm rounds
- 2 garlic cloves, crushed
- 1 tablespoon tomato purée
- 2 large boneless, skinless chicken breasts, sliced widthways into 5-mm strips
- 1 tablespoon dried oregano
- 200 g green lentils, rinsed
- 1.25 litres Dr. Hyman's Veggie-Bone Broth (page 128)
- 1 small cauliflower, trimmed
- 1 tablespoon sea salt
- 50 g toasted almonds, coarsely chopped

Warm the coconut oil in a large saucepan over a medium heat until melted. Add the onion, celery and carrots and cook, stirring occasionally, until the vegetables have softened, 4 to 5 minutes. Stir in the garlic and tomato purée and cook until fragrant and well combined, 2 to 3 minutes. Add the chicken, oregano, lentils and stock and stir to combine. Bring to a simmer, then cover and cook gently for 30 minutes, stirring occasionally, until the lentils are just shy of tender.

Meanwhile, use a paring knife to cut off the cauliflower florets, discarding the large central core. Cut the florets into 2.5-cm pieces.

Add the cauliflower to the pan, stir to combine, and continue to cook, covered, until the cauliflower and lentils are tender, about 15 minutes.

Stir in the salt and serve, sprinkling each portion with some of the chopped almonds.

Nutritional analysis per serving: Calories: 685, Fat: 34 g, Saturated Fat: 11 g, Cholesterol: 42 mg, Fiber: 41 g, Protein: 35 g, Carbohydrates: 80 g, Sodium: 734 mg

CREAMY FENNEL AND MUSHROOM SOUP

Traditionally used in Mediterranean cuisine, fennel is a feathery-leaved bulb with an aniseed flavor. Ancient medicine used it for an assortment of ailments, including upset stomachs and congestion. Blended with healing mushrooms, this soup will warm you up on a cold day or help soothe any symptoms of a cold.

Serves: 4
Prep tme: 20 minutes
Cook time: 40 minutes

- 1 large leek
- 1 large fennel bulb
- 5 large portobello mushrooms
- 1 tablespoon Ghee (page 279)
- 1 teaspoon sea salt
- 3 garlic cloves, crushed
- 250 ml dry white wine
- 750 ml unsweetened almond milk
- leaves from 1 large thyme sprig, well chopped (about 1 teaspoon)
- ¼ teaspoon freshly ground black pepper
- 1 tablespoon extra-virgin olive oil

Cut the root and green parts off the leek, then slice the white section in half lengthways and rinse under running water to remove any dirt that may have collected inside. Cut the leek halves into 1-cm pieces and set aside.

Trim off the fennel fronds, reserving them for garnish, then cut the bulb into quarters. Cut out the core, then slice the bulb into thin strips and set aside.

Remove the stems from the mushrooms, then use a spoon to carefully scrape away the gills, which are often full of dirt. Cut the caps into strips 5 mm thick.

Warm the ghee in a large saucepan over a medium heat until melted. Add the leeks and cook for 2 to 3 minutes, stirring occasionally. Stir in the fennel and continue cooking for another 2 to 3 minutes. Add the mushrooms, sprinkle in ½ teaspoon of the salt to help release their juices, and cook for 3 to 4 minutes, stirring occasionally and allowing them to brown slightly.

Stir in the garlic, cook until fragrant (about 45 seconds), then pour in the wine. Turn up the heat to medium-high and allow the wine to reduce by half. Pour in 500 ml of the almond milk, lower the heat back to medium, and simmer for 20 minutes.

Purée the contents of the pan in a blender, filling it no more more than half full, as hot liquids expand when blending. Cover the lid with a folded tea towel and hold it down as you blend, starting at low speed and gradually increasing to high. Slowly add the remaining almond milk as you are blending to thin the soup.

Return the soup to the pan and cook over a low heat for 2 minutes. Stir in the thyme and season the soup with the remaining salt and the pepper.

Ladle into bowls and serve garnished with a few chopped fennel fronds and a drizzle of the olive oil.

Nutritional analysis per serving: *Calories: 223, Fat: 9 g, Saturated Fat: 3 g, Cholesterol: 0 mg, Fiber: 5 g, Protein: 21 g, Carbohydrates: 14 g, Sodium: 612 mg*

10

Vegetables (Side Dishes and Main Dishes)

Savory Coconut Pancakes

These lightly spicy pancakes are quick and easy to make. Serve them topped with Shredded Chicken (page 201), with a savory cashew cream, or simply with grass-fed butter.

Makes: 12 tiny (2.5-cm) pancakes
Prep time: 10 minutes
Cook time: 10 minutes

- 4 large eggs
- 25 g coconut flour
- 1 teaspoon sea salt
- 1 teaspoon baking powder
- 1 teaspoon ground cumin
- 2 tablespoons roughly chopped fresh coriander
- ¼ teaspoon chipotle powder
- Ghee (page 279), for greasing

Crack the eggs into a large bowl and whisk gently. Add the coconut flour, salt, baking powder, cumin, coriander, chipotle powder and 2 tablespoons filtered water and whisk to combine. Let the batter stand for 5 minutes.

Warm 1 tablespoon ghee in a 20-cm frying pan over a medium heat until melted. Pour 2-tablespoon amounts of batter into the frying pan, forming as many 2.5-cm pancakes as will comfortably fit, and cook for 2 minutes. Use a metal spatula to flip them over, and continue to cook until they are slightly firm to the touch, about 1 more minute. Transfer the pancakes to a large plate. Grease the frying pan with more ghee and use the remaining batter to make more pancakes.

Serve warm or at room temperature.

Nutritional analysis per serving (3 pancakes): *Calories: 240, Fat: 21 g, Saturated Fat: 12 g, Cholesterol: 185 mg, Fiber: 3 g, Protein: 7 g, Carbohydrates: 5 g, Sodium: 523 mg*

WHITE BEAN PURÉE WITH ROSEMARY

PEGAN DIET

Silky smooth and seasoned with fresh rosemary, this simple bean purée is a great side dish to roasted vegetables and grilled chicken, lamb or beef. Although they may not agree with everyone, white beans contain essential nutrients and fiber that can improve cholesterol profiles, so feel free to try this purée after completing the twenty-one-day plan.

Makes: 500 g
Prep time: 15 minutes, plus soaking time
Cook time: 30 minutes

- 200 g dried cannellini beans
- 1 tablespoon apple cider vinegar
- 1 tablespoon Ghee (page 279)
- 1 small onion, thinly sliced
- 3 garlic cloves, crushed
- 750 ml chicken stock
- 1 bay leaf
- 2 tablespoons unsalted, grass-fed butter
- leaves from a 10-cm rosemary sprig, finely chopped
- 1 teaspoon sea salt
- ½ teaspoon freshly ground black pepper

Put the cannellini beans in a bowl, add the vinegar and cover with 1 litre warm filtered water. Set aside to soak at room temperature for at least 8 hours or up to 12 hours.

Drain the beans in a colander, rinse well and set aside.

Warm the ghee in a large saucepan over a medium heat until melted. Add the onion and cook, stirring occasionally, until softened and translucent, 3 to 4 minutes. Stir in the garlic and cook until fragrant, about 1 minute, then add the beans, 500 ml of the chicken stock and the bay leaf. Bring to a simmer, cover partially, and cook gently until the beans are very tender, 20 to 25 minutes.

Discard the bay leaf. Transfer a batch of beans and their cooking liquid to a blender, pour in some of the remaining stock and add the butter. Do not fill the blender more than halfway, as hot liquids expand when blending. Cover the lid with a folded tea towel and hold it down as you blend, starting at low speed and gradually increasing to high. Blend until smooth and creamy, about 45 seconds.

Return the purée to the saucepan and stir in the rosemary, salt and pepper. Warm over a low heat, stirring occasionally, until heated through. Serve.

Nutritional analysis per serving (125 g): *Calories: 279, Fat: 11 g, Saturated Fat: 6 g, Cholesterol: 71 mg, Fiber: 10 g, Protein: 12 g, Carbohydrates: 1 g, Sodium: 788 mg*

Italian Marinated Vegetables

This recipe features an assortment of delicious veggies and is a perfect side dish to just about any meal.

Serves: 4
Prep time: 20 minutes, plus chiling time

- 2 large carrots, scrubbed and trimmed
- 1 large fennel bulb, trimmed
- 1 small shallot, peeled
- 1 large broccoli head, stems peeled and cut into 5-mm rounds, florets cut into 2.5-cm pieces
- 2 tablespoons extra-virgin olive oil
- 4 tablespoons apple cider vinegar
- 4 tablespoons fresh lemon juice
- 2 tablespoons dulse flakes
- ½ tablespoon Dijon mustard
- 1 tablespoon nutritional yeast
- 1 teaspoon dried thyme
- 1 teaspoon dried oregano
- 1 teaspoon onion powder
- ½ teaspoon garlic powder
- ¼ teaspoon freshly ground black pepper

Use a mandoline or chef's knife to slice the carrots into 3-mm rounds (about the thickness of a £1 coin). Slice the fennel across the grain into 3-mm pieces, then slice the shallot into 3-mm rounds. Place the sliced vegetables in a large bowl along with the broccoli.

Put all the remaining ingredients in a separate bowl and whisk until well combined. Pour this dressing over the vegetables and toss until evenly coated. Cover and refrigerate for at least 20 minutes, or up to 8 hours.

Nutritional analysis per serving: *Calories: 256, Fat: 21 g, Saturated Fat: 3 g, Cholesterol: 0 mg, Fiber: 7 g, Protein: 5 g, Carbohydrates: 15 g, Sodium: 175 mg*

Confetti Vegetable Slaw with Tahini Dressing

Tahini is filled with vitamins and minerals that promote healthy cell growth, and it's also a great source of protein and healthy fat. Here it is mixed with phytonutrient-rich veggies to make a side dish that is the perfect accompaniment to any main course.

Serves: 4
Prep time: 20 minutes

- 1 large carrot, scrubbed
- 2 large beetroot, peeled
- 1 large watermelon radish (or regular radish), peeled
- 1 turnip, peeled
- 115 g unsalted tahini
- 4 tablespoons fresh lemon juice
- 3 garlic cloves
- 1 teaspoon sea salt
- 50 g fresh parsley leaves, roughly chopped
- 2 spring onions, thinly sliced
- 10 g toasted unsalted pumpkin seeds

Using the large holes of a box grater or a food processor fitted with the medium shredding disc, grate the carrot, beetroot, radish and turnip. Transfer them all to a large bowl.

Place the tahini, lemon juice, garlic, salt and 250 ml filtered water in a blender and blend on high speed until well combined. Transfer this dressing to a small bowl, then stir in the parsley and spring onions.

Pour the dressing over the vegetables and stir until evenly coated. Sprinkle with the pumpkin seeds and serve.

Nutritional analysis per serving: *Calories: 275, Fat: 20 g, Saturated Fat: 5 g, Cholesterol: 0 mg, Fiber: 7 g, Protein: 9 g, Carbohydrates: 19 g, Sodium: 686 mg*

RED CABBAGE SLAW WITH CUMIN

Everyone needs a go-to recipe for slaw, and this cumin-spiked version is the one I always turn to. It's especially good with grilled chicken or fish.

Serves: 4
Prep time: 15 minutes, plus marinating time

- 1 small red cabbage, finely shredded
- 2 sweet red peppers, seeded and thinly sliced
- 1 large carrot, scrubbed and grated
- 2 large tomatoes, cored and finely diced
- 1 bunch parsley, stemmed and roughly chopped
- 1 tablespoon cumin seed
- 4 tablespoons extra-virgin olive oil
- 1½ tablespoons apple cider vinegar
- 1 teaspoon sea salt

Place all the ingredients in a large bowl and toss well. Leave to stand for 10 to 15 minutes at room temperature so that the flavors will mingle. Serve.

Nutritional analysis per serving: *Calories: 220, Fat: 14 g, Saturated Fat: 2 g, Cholesterol: 0 mg, Fiber: 6 g, Protein: 4 g, Carbohydrates: 22 g, Sodium: 514 mg*

GINGER-TURMERIC CHINESE CABBAGE

Turmeric is a healing spice known for its anti-inflammatory properties. I make sure to use it whenever I have a cold or feel that my immune system needs a boost. Pair this dish with a side of bone broth for an extra-healing meal.

Serves: 4
Prep time: 5 minutes
Cook time: 10 minutes

- 2 tablespoons Ghee (page 279) or avocado oil
- 1 small head Chinese cabbage, shredded
- 2.5-cm piece fresh ginger, peeled and grated
- ½ teaspoon ground turmeric
- ¼ teaspoon freshly ground black pepper
- 1 tablespoon low-sodium, wheat-free tamari
- 1 tablespoon rice vinegar

Warm the ghee in a 25-cm frying pan over a medium-high heat until shimmering. Add the cabbage and cook, tossing continuously, until wilted and the volume has reduced by about half, 2 to 3 minutes. Add the ginger, turmeric and pepper and stir to combine. Drizzle in the tamari and vinegar, toss to incorporate, and serve.

Nutritional analysis per serving: *Calories: 138, Fat: 10 g, Saturated Fat: 5 g, Cholesterol: 0 mg, Fiber: 0 g, Protein: 5 g, Carbohydrates: 11 g, Sodium: 276 mg*

Cauliflower "Rice" with Spring Onions

You won't miss regular rice with this veggie alternative. Cauliflower "rice" will quickly become a staple recipe in your collection. It's easy to prepare and cooks more quickly than actual rice.

Serves: 4
Prep time: 5 minutes
Cook time: 10 minutes

- 1 cauliflower, trimmed
- 2 tablespoons extra-virgin olive oil
- 1 teaspoon sea salt
- 3 spring onions, thinly sliced

Using a chef's knife, cut the cauliflower in half, then use a paring knife to cut off the florets. Cut the florets and the core into roughly 1-cm pieces.

Pulse about 200 g of the cauliflower pieces in a food processor until broken down into fine bits that resemble grains of rice, 6 to 8 two–second pulses. Transfer to a large bowl and repeat with the remaining cauliflower.

Warm the olive oil in a 25-cm frying pan over a medium–high heat until shimmering. Add the cauliflower and cook, stirring frequently, until tender, 4 to 5 minutes. Stir in the salt and spring onions and serve.

Nutritional analysis per serving: *Calories: 92, Fat: 7 g, Saturated Fat: 1 g, Cholesterol: 0 mg, Fiber: 3 g, Protein: 3 g, Carbohydrates: 7 g, Sodium: 478 mg*

CURRIED CAULIFLOWER WITH PEAS AND MINT

This flavorful curried cauliflower dish is the perfect accompaniment to slow-cooked lamb, grilled chicken, or even grilled tofu.

Serves: 4
Prep time: 10 minutes
Cook time: 15 minutes

- 1 large cauliflower, trimmed
- 2 tablespoons Ghee (page 279)
- 1 small red onion, thinly sliced
- 1 tablespoon curry powder
- 1 teaspoon sea salt
- 65 ml chicken or vegetable stock
- 120 g fresh or defrosted frozen peas
- 35 g dried currants
- 35 g unsalted roasted cashews
- 2 tablespoons julienned fresh mint leaves
- juice of 1 lemon

Using a paring knife, cut the florets off the cauliflower and discard the large core. Cut the florets into 2.5-cm pieces.

Warm the ghee oil in a large frying pan over a medium-high heat until melted. Add the onion and cook, stirring occasionally, until softened, 2 to 3 minutes. Add the cauliflower, curry powder and salt, toss to combine, and cook for 2 minutes. Pour in the stock, then cover and cook until the cauliflower is tender, 3 to 4 minutes.

Add the peas to the cauliflower and stir to combine. Fold in the currants, cashews, mint, and lemon juice and serve.

Peas not cooked or defrosted?

Nutritional analysis per serving: *Calories: 213, Fat: 12 g, Saturated Fat: 5 g, Cholesterol: 0 mg, Fiber: 6 g, Protein: 7 g, Carbohydrates: 24 g, Sodium: 697 mg*

Asparagus with Toasted Hazelnuts and Lemon

Asparagus is packed with glutathione, the mother of all antioxidants and a powerful detoxifier that has been shown to help prevent ageing, cancer, heart disease and dementia. Serve this side dish alongside roasted fish, grilled tofu or seared steak.

Serves: 4
Prep time: 10 minutes
Cook time: 20 minutes

- 1 teaspoon sea salt
- 900 g asparagus, trimmed
- 2 tablespoons unsalted, grass-fed butter
- 75 g hazelnuts, coarsely chopped
- 1 large shallot, sliced into 5-mm rounds
- grated zest and juice of 1 lemon
- ¼ teaspoon freshly ground black pepper

Pour 750 ml filtered water into a large saucepan and bring to a simmer over a medium–high heat. Meanwhile, fill a large bowl with iced water.

Add ½ teaspoon of the salt and the asparagus to the simmering water and cook until the spears are tender, 3 to 4 minutes. Drain immediately and transfer the asparagus to the iced water to stop the cooking. Once it has chilled, drain again and set aside.

Warm the butter in a large frying pan over a medium heat until melted. Add the hazelnuts and shallot and cook, stirring occasionally, until the shallot softens and the hazelnuts are golden brown, about 3 minutes. Add the asparagus and toss to combine. Sprinkle in the lemon zest and juice along with the remaining salt and pepper. Toss again to combine and cook just until the asparagus is heated through, 30 to 60 seconds. Transfer to a platter and serve.

Nutritional analysis per serving: *Calories: 186, Fat: 15 g, Saturated Fat: 4 g, Cholesterol: 15 mg, Fiber: 6 g, Protein: 6 g, Carbohydrates: 12 g, Sodium: 565 mg*

GARLIC-STEAMED CHARD

Here the slightly bitter flavour of chard is complemented with lots of garlic and dried red chili flakes. Other types of greens, such as kale or broccoli, can be used if you wish.

Serves: 4
Prep time: 10 minutes
Cook time: 10 minutes

- 2 tablespoons extra-virgin olive oil
- 1 tablespoon unsalted, grass-fed butter
- 3 garlic cloves, thinly sliced
- 2 bunches chard, trimmed and cut into thirds
- ½ teaspoon dried red chili flakes
- 1 teaspoon sea salt

Warm the olive oil and butter in a 30-cm frying pan over a medium-high heat until the butter foams. Add the garlic and cook, stirring occasionally, until lightly browned, about 2 minutes. Add the chard, toss to coat with the fat, and pour in 125 ml filtered water. Cover and cook until tender, about 5 minutes.

Sprinkle the dried red chili flakes and salt over the chard, toss to combine, and serve.

Nutritional analysis per serving: *Calories: 180, Fat: 16 g, Saturated Fat: 4 g, Cholesterol: 8 mg, Fiber: 3 g, Protein: 4 g, Carbohydrates: 4 g, Sodium: 606 mg*

CREAMED TURMERIC CAVOLO NERO WITH RED PEPPERS

Here we have comfort food with a nutritional upgrade. Turmeric, an inflammation-fighting spice, pairs nicely with rich coconut cream. This simple dish is a unique and tasty way to enjoy 'black cabbage'.

Serves: 4
Prep time: 15 minutes
Cook time: 10 minutes

- 2 tablespoons extra-virgin olive oil
- 2 garlic cloves, thinly sliced
- 2 sweet red peppers, seeded and finely diced
- 2 bunches cavolo nero, stemmed and roughly chopped
- 65 ml full-fat coconut milk
- 1 teaspoon ground turmeric
- ½ teaspoon sea salt

Warm the olive oil in a 25-cm frying pan over a medium heat until shimmering. Stir in the garlic and cook until fragrant, about 30 seconds. Add the peppers and cook, stirring occasionally, until just beginning to soften, about 2 minutes. Add the cavolo nero, toss with tongs to combine, and pour in the coconut milk. Stir in the turmeric and salt, then cover and cook, stirring occasionally, until the cabbage is wilted, 2 to 3 minutes. Serve.

Nutritional analysis per serving: *Calories: 157, Fat: 8 g, Saturated Fat: 1 g, Cholesterol: 0 mg, Fiber: 3 g, Protein: 3 g, Carbohydrates: 12 g, Sodium: 307 mg*

BRAISED SPRING GREENS

Cabbage comes in many different varieties, but the best ones for this recipe come from loose-leaved heads, like spring greens. The benefits of consuming greens are numerous, but a notable one is lowered cholesterol. In this recipe the leaves are buttery and delicious.

Serves: 4
Prep time: 10 minutes
Cook time: 45 minutes

- 2 tablespoons Ghee (page 279)
- 1 large onion, thinly sliced
- 3 garlic cloves, crushed
- 900 g spring greens or loose-leaved cabbage, tough stems removed and leaves sliced
- 500 ml chicken or vegetable stock
- 1 teaspoon sea salt
- ¼ teaspoon freshly ground black pepper

Warm the ghee in a large saucepan over a medium heat until shimmering. Add the onion and cook, stirring occasionally, until slightly softened, about 2 minutes. Stir in the garlic and cook until fragrant, about 1 minute. Add the greens and cook, stirring to combine, for 1 minute. Pour in the stock and bring to a simmer. Cover and cook until the greens are tender, about 40 minutes.

Stir in the salt and pepper and serve the greens straight away.

Nutritional analysis per serving: *Calories: 135, Fat: 9 g, Saturated Fat: 5 g, Cholesterol: 4 mg, Fiber: 1 g, Protein: 4 g, Carbohydrates: 10 g, Sodium: 737 mg*

Celeriac Hash

Rich in vitamins A, C, K and E, as well as other nutrients, celeriac makes a fantastic mash that goes well with all sorts of main dishes. It's the best kind of 'healthfood'!

Serves: 4
Prep time: 10 minutes
Cook time: 20 minutes

- 1 to 2 tablespoons extra-virgin olive oil
- 1 tablespoon unsalted, grass-fed butter
- 2 large celeriac, peeled and finely diced
- 1 small onion, finely diced
- leaves from 2 rosemary sprigs, finely chopped
- 1 teaspoon sea salt
- ¼ teaspoon freshly ground black pepper

Warm 1 tablespoon of the olive oil and the butter in a large frying pan over a medium heat until the butter melts. Add the celeriac, toss to coat with the fat, and cook, stirring occasionally, until slightly softened, 7 to 8 minutes. Stir in the onion and continue to cook until the celeriac is tender, about 10 minutes, adding an additional 1 tablespoon oil if needed to prevent sticking.

Stir in the rosemary, salt and pepper and serve.

Nutritional analysis per serving: *Calories: 117, Fat: 10 g, Saturated Fat: 3 g, Cholesterol: 8 mg, Fiber: 3 g, Protein: 1 g, Carbohydrates: 5 g, Sodium: 442 mg*

Courgetti with Shiitake Mushrooms and Ume Vinegar

Umeboshi, also known simply as 'ume', are plum-like Japanese fruits that are traditionally preserved in salt. They have a long history of use as a digestive aid. The liquid that the fruits release during the salting process is referred to as 'ume vinegar', though it is not actually vinegar.

Serves: 4
Prep time: 10 minutes
Cook time: 10 minutes

- 2 large courgettes, ends trimmed
- 2 tablespoons sesame oil
- 2 garlic cloves, crushed
- 225 g shiitake mushrooms, stemmed and sliced into 5-mm strips
- 1 tablespoon ume vinegar
- 1 tablespoon toasted sesame oil
- 1 teaspoon dried red chili flakes
- 1 sheet nori, quartered and cut into thin strips

Using a vegetable peeler, or a spiralizer fitted with a shredder blade, cut the courgettes into spaghetti-like strands. Use kitchen shears to cut them into shorter lengths.

Warm the sesame oil in a 25-cm frying pan over a medium–high heat until shimmering. Add the garlic and mushrooms and cook, stirring frequently, until the mushrooms are softened and lightly browned, 3 to 4 minutes. Add the 'courgetti', vinegar, toasted sesame oil and red chili flakes and cook, tossing to combine, until the courgetti are just warmed through, about 3 minutes.

Divide the courgetti mixture between 4 plates. Sprinkle each portion with nori strips and serve.

Nutritional analysis per serving: *Calories: 161, Fat: 11 g, Saturated Fat: 2 g, Cholesterol: 0 mg, Fiber: 0 g, Protein: 3 g, Carbohydrates: 14 g, Sodium: 445 mg*

Stir-Fried Broccoli and Cabbage with Ginger-Avocado Sauce

Here's a vibrant stir-fry that can be made with whatever vegetables are fresh and in season. The rich and creamy avocado sauce is an unusual touch that adds great flavor and healthy fats to this meal.

Serves: 4
Prep time: 15 minutes
Cook time: 20 minutes

- 5-cm piece fresh ginger, peeled
- 2 avocados, stoned, peeled and cut into large chunks
- 2 tablespoons fresh lime juice
- ¼ teaspoon sea salt
- ¼ teaspoon freshly ground black pepper
- 200 ml cold filtered water
- 2 tablespoons coconut oil
- ¼ head cabbage (any kind), cored and shredded
- 1 small red onion, thinly sliced
- 2 garlic cloves, crushed
- 1 large head broccoli, stems peeled and cut into rounds 5 mm thick, florets cut into bite-sized pieces
- 60 g baby rocket
- 4 tablespoons toasted sesame seeds (optional)

To make the sauce, pulse the ginger in a food processor until minced. Add the avocados, lime juice, salt and pepper and process until smooth. With the machine running, add 125 ml of the water 1 to 2 tablespoons at a time until the sauce is thick and creamy. Transfer to a bowl, then cover and refrigerate until required.

Warm the sesame oil in a 25–cm frying pan over a medium heat until melted. Add the cabbage and onion and cook, stirring occasionally, until wilted and softened, 3 to 4 minutes. Stir in the garlic and cook until fragrant, about 1 minute. Add the broccoli, stir to combine, then pour in the remaining water. Cover and cook until the broccoli is tender, about 3 minutes.

Divide the rocket between 4 plates and top with the stir-fry. Spoon about 4 tablespoons of the sauce over each portion, sprinkle with a tablespoon of the sesame seeds, if using, and serve.

Nutritional analysis per serving: Calories: 357, Fat: 31 g, Saturated Fat: 9 g, Cholesterol: 0 mg, Fiber: 9 g, Protein: 6 g, Carbohydrates: 20 g, Sodium: 293 mg

GINGER-TAMARI BAKED TOFU AND MUSHROOMS

Tofu's neutral taste and ability to absorb flavors means you can infuse it with just about any seasonings you desire. Here it's marinated, along with earthy shiitake mushrooms, in Japanese staple ingredients for a deeply savory vegetarian main dish.

Serves: 4
Prep time: 15 minutes, plus marinating time
Cook time: 30 minutes

- 450 g non-GMO firm tofu, drained
- 450 g shiitake mushrooms, stemmed
- 2 tablespoons toasted sesame oil
- 1 tablespoon low-sodium, wheat-free tamari
- 2 tablespoons apple cider vinegar
- 1 tablespoon mirin
- 2 garlic cloves, crushed
- 2.5-cm piece fresh ginger, peeled and finely chopped
- 1 teaspoon dried red chili flakes
- 2 spring onions, thinly sliced

Place the tofu on a plate. Set another plate on top and weigh it down with 2 cans of food weighing a total of 800 g. Leave to stand at room temperature for 30 minutes.

Transfer the tofu to a chopping board and cut it into 8 equal cubes. Place in a non-metallic baking dish with the mushrooms.

Put the sesame oil in a bowl, add the tamari, vinegar, mirin, garlic, ginger and red chili flakes and stir to combine. Pour this mixture over the tofu and mushrooms and toss to coat. Cover and refrigerate for 1 to 24 hours, depending how much time you have.

Preheat the oven to 180°C/350°F/Gas 4. Line a baking sheet with baking parchment.

Remove the tofu and mushrooms from the marinade and place them in a single layer on the prepared baking sheet. Bake for 15 minutes, then flip them over and continue to bake until the tofu is lightly browned and the mushrooms are slightly crisp at the edges, about 15 more minutes.

Transfer the tofu and mushrooms to a platter. Top with the spring onions and serve.

Nutritional analysis per serving: *Calories: 247, Fat: 15 g, Saturated Fat: 4 g, Cholesterol: 0 mg, Fiber: 3 g, Protein: 18 g, Carbohydrates: 14 g, Sodium: 213 mg*

Baked Marinated Tempeh with Shiitake-Turnip-Chard Hash

If you've never tried tempeh (fermented tofu), this dish is a great introduction. Marinating and roasting the tempeh squares infuses them with bold, savory flavor that is complemented by the earthy vegetable hash. The marinade includes coconut aminos, a soya-free seasoning produced from the sap of the coconut tree. It's available online, but tamari can be used instead.

Serves: 4
Prep time: 20 minutes, plus marinating time
Cook time: 20 minutes

- 500 g organic, GMO-free tempeh, cut into 8 equal squares
- 60 ml extra-virgin olive oil
- 4 tablespoons coconut aminos or wheat-free tamari
- 2 tablespoons balsamic vinegar
- 2 tablespoons apple cider vinegar
- 2 tablespoons wholegrain mustard
- 4 garlic cloves, crushed
- ¼ teaspoon chipotle powder
- 2 tablespoons coconut oil
- 1 large turnip, peeled and finely diced
- 1 small red onion, finely chopped
- 10 large shiitake mushrooms, stemmed and sliced into thirds
- 4 large chard leaves, stemmed and cut into bite-sized pieces

Place the tempeh in a non-metallic baking dish. Put the olive oil in a bowl, add the coconut aminos, balsamic vinegar, cider vinegar, mustard, half the garlic and the chipotle powder and whisk together. Pour this mixture over the tempeh, then cover and gently shake the baking dish to coat the tempeh. Refrigerate for 8 to 24 hours, depending how much time you have, turning the tempeh pieces once or twice.

Preheat the oven to 180°C/350°F/Gas 4.

Uncover the tempeh and place the dish in the oven until the tempeh pieces are browned on the bottom, about 15 minutes.

Meanwhile, warm 1 tablespoon of the coconut oil in a 25-cm frying pan over a medium heat until melted. Add the turnip and onion and cook, stirring occasionally, until the turnip begins to soften, about 5 minutes. Add the mushrooms, the remaining coconut oil and garlic and cook, stirring occasionally, until the turnip is tender, 8 to 10 minutes. Stir in the chard and cook until the leaves are wilted.

Divide the vegetable hash between 4 plates, then top each portion with 2 pieces of tempeh. Drizzle the marinade remaining in the baking dish over the top and serve.

Nutritional analysis per serving: *Calories: 563, Fat: 42 g, Saturated Fat: 11 g, Cholesterol: 0 mg, Fiber: 12 g, Protein: 25 g, Carbohydrates: 29 g, Sodium: 1065 mg*

Tempeh and Sweet Peppers with Tomato and Cardamom

Cardamom is a warm, fragrant spice from a plant native to India, and it's commonly used in that country's cuisine. This dish, paired with Cauliflower "Rice" with Spring onions (page 156), makes a great vegetarian meal.

Serves: 4
Prep time: 10 minutes
Cook time: 20 minutes

- 1 tablespoon Ghee (page 279)
- 225 g organic, non-GMO tempeh, cut into 1-cm chunks
- 1 large red onion, finely diced
- 1 sweet red pepper, seeded and finely diced
- 1 sweet green pepper, seeded and finely diced
- 2 teaspoons ground cardamom
- 2 garlic cloves, crushed
- 260 g tomato purée
- 250 ml vegetable stock or filtered water
- ½ teaspoon sea salt
- 8 g fresh coriander leaves, roughly chopped

Warm the ghee in a large frying pan over a medium heat until melted. Add the tempeh and onion, toss to combine, and cook until the onion begins to soften, 2 to 3 minutes. Add the peppers and cook, stirring occasionally, until they begin to soften, 2 to 3 minutes. Stir in the cardamom and garlic and cook until fragrant, about 1 minute. Add the tomato purée and stock and stir to combine. Cover and simmer, stirring occasionally, until all the liquid has been absorbed, 15 to 20 minutes.

Stir in the salt and coriander and serve.

Nutritional analysis per serving: *Calories: 186, Fat: 7 g, Saturated Fat: 3 g, Cholesterol: 0 mg, Fiber: 8 g, Protein: 13 g, Carbohydrates: 19 g, Sodium: 333 mg*

TEMPEH, VEGETABLE AND KELP NOODLE STIR-FRY

Kelp noodles are a great alternative to wheat and rice noodles.

Serves: 4
Prep time: 20 minutes
Cook time: 10 minutes

- 3 tablespoons sesame oil
- 225 g organic, non-GMO tempeh, cut into eighths
- 1 small onion, thinly sliced
- 1 large carrot, scrubbed and thinly sliced diagonally
- 200 g broccoli florets, cut into 2.5-cm pieces
- 150 g thinly sliced cavolo nero

- 2.5-cm piece fresh ginger, peeled and finely chopped
- 125 ml chicken or vegetable stock
- 3 tablespoons wheat-free tamari
- 450 g kelp noodles, cut into 10-cm lengths and rinsed
- 1 bunch spring onions, green parts only, thinly sliced

Warm 1 tablespoon of the sesame oil in a 25-cm frying pan over a medium-high heat until shimmering. Add the tempeh and cook until browned, about 2 minutes, then flip and cook for an additional 1 to 2 minutes. Transfer to a plate. Add the remaining 2 tablespoons sesame oil to the pan and heat until shimmering. Add the onion, carrot, broccoli and cavolo nero and cook, stirring occasionally, until the vegetables are slightly softened, 3 to 4 minutes.

Meanwhile, bring 1 litre filtered water to a simmer in a saucepan. Add the kelp noodles and cook just until heated through, about 3 minutes, then drain.

Stir the ginger, stock, tamari and tempeh into the vegetable mixture, then remove the pan from the heat. Add the noodles to the frying pan, return to a medium-high heat, and toss until well combined. Mix in the spring onion greens and serve.

Nutritional analysis per serving: *Calories: 265, Fat: 14 g, Saturated Fat: 2 g, Cholesterol: 1 mg, Fiber: 7 g, Protein: 15 g, Carbohydrates: 20 g, Sodium: 680 mg*

11

Seafood

TAMARI AND ORANGE-MARINATED COD WITH BOK CHOY

PEGAN DIET

Here's a simple but wholesome fish and vegetable dish that requires minimal prep and cooks in only 15 minutes, making it a perfect weeknight meal.

Serves: 4
Prep time: 10 minutes, plus marinating time
Cook time: 15 minutes

- 2 tablespoons low-sodium, wheat-free tamari
- 1 tablespoon fish sauce
- 1 tablespoon rice vinegar
- 4 tablespoons fresh orange juice
- 2.5-cm piece fresh ginger, peeled and crushed
- 4 x 100-g cod fillets
- 1 tablespoon sesame oil
- 2 garlic cloves, crushed
- 1 large head bok choy, cut widthways into 2.5-cm pieces, rinsed and drained

Put 1 tablespoon of the tamari in a 20-cm non-metallic baking dish, add the fish sauce, vinegar, orange juice and ginger and stir together. Add the cod fillets in a single layer and flip them over several times to coat well with the marinade. Cover and refrigerate for 30 minutes.

Preheat the oven to 180°C/350°F/Gas 4. Transfer the fish to a clean baking dish and bake until the flesh is firm and flakes easily, about 8 minutes.

Meanwhile, warm the sesame oil in a 25-cm frying pan over a medium-high heat until shimmering. Add the garlic and cook, stirring frequently, until lightly browned, about 1 minute. Stir in the bok choy, then add 4 tablespoons filtered water and the remaining tamari. Cover and cook until the stems are al dente, 2 to 3 minutes. Divide the bok choy between 4 plates, and top with a cod fillet.

Nutritional analysis per serving: *Calories: 182, Fat: 5 g, Saturated Fat: 1 g, Cholesterol: 0 mg, Fiber: 0 g, Protein: 27 g, Carbohydrates: 5 g, Sodium: 791 mg*

Baked Haddock with Fennel-Cauliflower Purée

Here is a simple but elegant dish. The fennel imparts a sweet and earthy flavor to the cauliflower, and a herbal aroma to the fish.

Serves: 4
Prep time: 20 minutes
Cook time: 20 minutes

- 1 cauliflower, trimmed
- 2 tablespoons extra-virgin olive oil
- 3 tablespoons unsalted, grass-fed butter
- 1 large leek, white section halved lengthways, rinsed well and thinly sliced
- 1 large fennel bulb, fronds reserved, bulb cut in half, cored and roughly chopped
- 2 garlic cloves, crushed
- 250 ml chicken stock
- 2 x 225-g skinless haddock fillets
- 1 teaspoon sea salt
- ½ teaspoon freshly ground black pepper

Preheat the oven to 180°C/350°F/Gas 4.

Cut the cauliflower in half, then use a paring knife to cut off the florets. Discard the large core and cut the florets into roughly 2.5-cm pieces.

Warm 1 tablespoon of the olive oil and 1 tablespoon of the butter in a large saucepan over a medium heat until the butter melts. Add the leek and fennel and cook, stirring occasionally, until softened but not at all browned, about 5 minutes. Stir in the garlic and cook until fragrant, about 2–3 minutes. Add the cauliflower and stir to combine. Pour in the stock, then cover and simmer, stirring occasionally, until the vegetables are completely tender, about 10 minutes.

Meanwhile, lay half the fennel fronds in a baking tin. Place the fish on top, drizzle with the remaining 1 tablespoon olive oil, and sprinkle with ½ teaspoon of the salt and ¼ teaspoon of the pepper. Top the fillets with the remaining fennel fronds. Bake the fish until just firm to the touch and opaque throughout, 10 to 12 minutes. Remove from the oven and carefully scrape away the fennel fronds on top. Cut each fillet in half widthways.

When the vegetables are tender, transfer them to a food processor. Add the remaining butter, salt and pepper and purée until smooth, scraping down the bowl as needed, about 1 minute. Return the purée to the pan and cover to keep warm.

Divide the vegetable purée between 4 plates and top each portion with a piece of fish. Serve.

Nutritional analysis per serving: *Calories: 346, Fat: 18 g, Saturated Fat: 7 g, Cholesterol: 119 mg, Fiber: 4 g, Protein: 33 g, Carbohydrates: 13 g, Sodium: 860 mg*

LEMON-BAKED SOLE WITH STEWED SUMMER SQUASH

Sole is a delicate white fish that pairs well with a wide range of ingredients. Here it is combined with fresh summer squash, herbs and rocket for a light, healthful meal.

Serves: 4
Prep time: 20 minutes
Cook time: 25 minutes

- 3 tablespoons extra-virgin olive oil
- 4 x 175-g skinless sole or flounder fillets
- 2 teaspoons chopped fresh thyme
- ½ teaspoon sea salt
- ½ teaspoon freshly ground black pepper
- ½ small red onion, very thinly sliced
- 1 lemon, thinly sliced
- 1 tablespoon Ghee (page 279)
- 2 yellow summer squash, cut into rounds 5 mm thick
- 3 garlic cloves, crushed
- 2 teaspoons dried oregano
- 1 large tomato, roughly chopped
- 40 g baby rocket

Preheat the oven to 180°C/350°F/Gas 4.

Drizzle 1 tablespoon of the olive oil into a baking dish large enough to hold the fish in a single layer. Place the fillets in it and sprinkle evenly with the thyme, a pinch of salt and ¼ teaspoon of the pepper. Scatter the onion slices over the top, then drizzle with 1 tablespoon of the remaining olive oil. Arrange the lemon slices over the fillets, then set aside.

Warm the remaining olive oil and the ghee in a 30-cm frying pan over a medium-high heat until shimmering. Add the squash, toss gently and cook, stirring occasionally, until it begins to soften, about 3 minutes. Stir in the garlic, oregano and remaining salt.

Place the fish in the oven and bake until the fillets are just firm to the touch and opaque throughout, 6 to 8 minutes. Meanwhile, continue cooking the squash, stirring occasionally, until tender.

After removing the fish from the oven, add the tomato to the squash, toss to combine, and cook until the tomato is just warmed through, 1 to 2 minutes.

Divide the rocket between 4 plates and spoon the squash mixture on top. Carefully place a fish fillet, including the onion and lemon slices, on each portion of squash and serve.

Nutritional analysis per serving: *Calories: 445, Fat: 33 g, Saturated Fat: 7 g, Cholesterol: 93 mg, Fiber: 3 g, Protein: 31 g, Carbohydrates: 7 g, Sodium: 320 mg*

Coconut Sole with Black Beans and Spinach

PEGAN DIET

Everyone should have a few healthful-one-pot meals like this one in his or her repertoire for those days when dinner needs to be on the table in an instant. This delicious Mexican-influenced dish is loaded with flavor but can be prepared in only 20 minutes.

Serves: 4
Prep time: 5 minutes
Cook time: 15 minutes

- 2 tablespoons coconut oil
- 1 large onion, thinly sliced
- 1 x 400-g can black beans, rinsed and drained
- 1 teaspoon ground cumin
- 1 teaspoon ground coriander
- ¾ teaspoon sea salt
- 4 tablespoons full-fat coconut milk
- 350 g baby spinach
- 4 x 100-g skinless sole or flounder fillets
- juice of ½ lime

Warm the coconut oil in a 25-cm frying pan over a medium heat until melted. Add the onion and cook, stirring occasionally, until softened, 2 to 3 minutes. Add the beans, cumin, coriander and a pinch of the salt and stir to combine. Pour in the coconut milk and bring to a simmer. Scatter the spinach in an even layer in the pan and use your hands to slightly flatten the leaves. Lay the fish in a single layer on top of the spinach, sprinkle the fillets with the remaining salt, and squeeze the lime juice over the top. Cover and cook until the fish is opaque throughout, 4 to 5 minutes.

Divide the fish, spinach and bean mixture between 4 plates and serve.

Nutritional analysis per serving: *Calories: 309, Fat: 11 g, Saturated Fat: 9 g, Cholesterol: 62 mg, Fiber: 7 g, Protein: 27 g, Carbohydrates: 24 g, Sodium: 855 mg*

Sautéed Perch with Tomato-Mango Salsa

PEGAN DIET

The colorful, tangy-sweet salsa is the perfect pairing for perch's mild flavor.

Serves: 4
Prep time: 20 minutes
Cook time: 15 minutes

- 1 mango, peeled and cut into 5-mm dice
- 1 large tomato, cut into 5-mm dice
- 5 g fresh coriander leaves, roughly chopped
- grated zest and juice of 1 lime
- 4 tablespoons extra-virgin olive oil
- 1 small jalapeño chili, seeded and finely chopped
- 8 x 50-g skin-on perch fillets
- 1 teaspoon sea salt
- 1 teaspoon ground cumin
- ¼ teaspoon freshly ground black pepper
- 2 tablespoons Ghee (page 279)

Put the mango in a bowl with the tomato, coriander, lime zest and juice, olive oil and chili. Mix well, then leave to stand so that the flavors can mingle while you prepare the fish.

Season the perch fillets with the salt, cumin and pepper. Warm the ghee in a large frying pan over a medium-high heat until shimmering. Lay the fillets flesh side down in a single layer in the frying pan and cook until half-done, about 3 minutes. Using a metal spatula, flip them over, then turn off the heat and let the fish finish cooking in the pan's residual heat, about 2 minutes.

Place 2 fillets on each serving plate. Top each portion with the salsa and serve.

Nutritional analysis per serving: *Calories: 538, Fat: 29 g, Saturated Fat: 8 g, Cholesterol: 111 mg, Fiber: 6 g, Protein: 47 g, Carbohydrates: 25 g, Sodium: 1377 mg*

Baked Halibut with Butternut Squash-Carrot Purée

In addition to being amazingly delicious, this simple dish is incredibly good for you. Butternut squash is rich in fiber, antioxidants and phytonutrients, while carrots are loaded with beta-carotene, and halibut is rich in omega-3 fats.

Serves: 4
Prep time: 10 minutes
Cook time: 20 minutes

- 2 tablespoons coconut oil
- 1 spring onion, thinly sliced
- 2 carrots, scrubbed and cut into 2.5-cm pieces
- 1 small butternut squash, peeled, seeded and cut into 2.5-cm cubes
- 3 tablespoons coconut butter
- 2 tablespoons apple cider vinegar
- 2 teaspoons sea salt
- 2 teaspoons chopped fresh thyme
- 2 teaspoons paprika
- ¼ teaspoon freshly ground black pepper
- 750 g halibut fillets (or other lean white fish, such as haddock or cod)
- 2 tablespoons extra-virgin olive oil

Preheat the oven to 180°C/350°F/Gas 4.

Warm the coconut oil in a large saucepan over a medium heat until melted. Add the spring onion and cook, stirring occasionally, until softened, about 2 minutes. Add the carrots and butternut squash, stir to combine, then pour in 125 ml filtered water. Cover and cook until the vegetables are completely tender, 6 to 7 minutes.

Transfer the vegetables to a food processor and pulse a few times to break down the pieces. Add the coconut butter, vinegar and 1 teaspoon of the salt and process until the mixture has the consistency of mashed potatoes, about 30 seconds. Return the purée to the saucepan and cover to keep warm.

Put the thyme, paprika, pepper and remaining salt in a small bowl and stir together. Coat the fish fillets all over with the olive oil, then rub with the thyme mixture. Place the fish in a single layer in a baking dish and bake until opaque throughout, 8 to 10 minutes.

Divide the vegetable purée between 4 plates, top each portion with a piece of fish, and serve.

Nutritional analysis per serving: Calories: 432, Fat: 32 g, Saturated Fat: 20 g, Cholesterol: 0 mg, Fiber: 4 g, Protein: 28 g, Carbohydrates: 11 g, Sodium: 677 mg

ARCTIC CHAR WITH CHARD AND MUSTARD VINAIGRETTE

According to seafood watch lists, Arctic char is sustainable and therefore a good choice for eco-conscious consumers. The pink-fleshed cold-water fish can be prepared in the same ways as salmon, its close relative. Chard contains numerous polyphenols, which have been shown to help regulate blood sugar, and that's just one of the vegetable's many benefits.

Serves: 4
Prep time: 15 minutes
Cook time: 15 minutes

- 6 tablspoons extra-virgin olive oil
- 2 tablespoons apple cider vinegar
- 1½ tablespoons wholegrain mustard
- 4 x 100-g skin-on Arctic char fillets
- 1 teaspoon sea salt, plus an extra pinch
- ½ teaspoon freshly ground black pepper
- 1 tablespoon Ghee (page 279)
- 300 g chard, stemmed and leaves cut into bite-sized pieces
- slice of lemon and sprinkle of fresh parsley, to garnish (optional)

To make the mustard vinaigrette, put 4 tablespoons of the olive oil in a small bowl, add the vinegar and mustard and whisk together. Set aside.

Season the fish with the teaspoon of salt and the pepper. Warm the ghee in a large, heavy-based frying pan over a medium-high heat until shimmering. Carefully place the fish flesh side down in the pan and cook until half-done, about 4 minutes. Using a metal spatula, flip the fish over, then turn off the heat and let the fish finish cooking in the pan's residual heat, about 2 minutes.

Meanwhile, warm the remaining olive oil in a separate large frying pan over a medium-high heat until shimmering. Add the chard and a pinch of salt. Using tongs, toss the chard and cook until completely wilted, about 3 minutes.

Divide the chard between 4 plates and top each portion with a fish fillet. Whisk the vinaigrette to recombine, then drizzle it over the chard and fish. Garnishe with the lemon and parsley, if using, and serve.

Nutritional analysis per serving: *Calories: 405, Fat: 30 g, Saturated Fat: 9 g, Cholesterol: 32 mg, Fiber: 1 g, Protein: 25 g, Carbohydrates: 1 g, Sodium: 854 mg*

DILL BUTTER-BAKED SALMON WITH BEETROOT AND ROASTED PEPPER SALAD

When it comes to fish, wild salmon is my top choice because it contains large amounts of omega-3 fatty acids and is widely regarded as a superfood. A 100-g piece of baked or grilled salmon contains at least 2 g of omega-3 fats! So if you're looking to add more omega-3s to your diet, try this buttery baked salmon with a delicious beetroot salad accompaniment. I prefer the flavor and texture of salmon when the center of the fillet is still slightly translucent, but you can cook the fillets until done to your liking.

Serves: 4
Prep time: 10 minutes
Cook time: 20 minutes

- 3 large beetroot, peeled and finely diced
- 2 large roasted red peppers from a jar, sliced into thin strips
- 1 shallot, sliced into thin rounds
- 1 tablespoon roughly chopped fresh parsley leaves
- 1½ tablespoons balsamic vinegar
- 3 tablespoons extra-virgin olive oil
- ½ teaspoon sea salt
- ½ teaspoon freshly ground black pepper
- 4 x 100-g wild salmon fillets
- 8 tablespoons unsalted, grass-fed butter, at room temperature
- 1 tablespoon roughly chopped fresh dill leaves
- 1 lemon, halved and seeded

Preheat the oven to 180°C/350°F/Gas 4.

Place the beetroot in a saucepan and cover with filtered water. Bring to the boil over a high heat, then simmer until the beetroot are tender, about 10 minutes. Drain, then submerge in a bowl of cold water until cooled, and drain again.

Place the beetroot in a bowl with the roasted peppers, shallot, parsley, vinegar, olive oil, salt and ¼ teaspoon of the pepper. Mix well, then set aside.

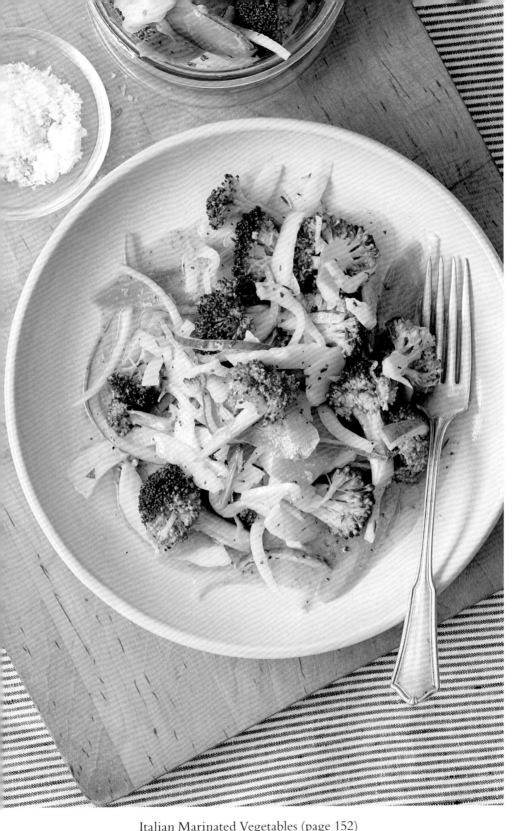

Italian Marinated Vegetables (page 152)

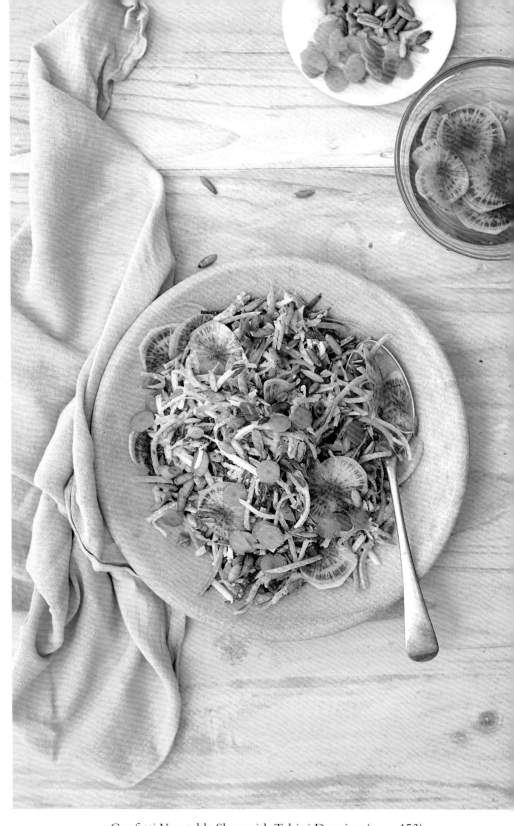

Confetti Vegetable Slaw with Tahini Dressing (page 153)

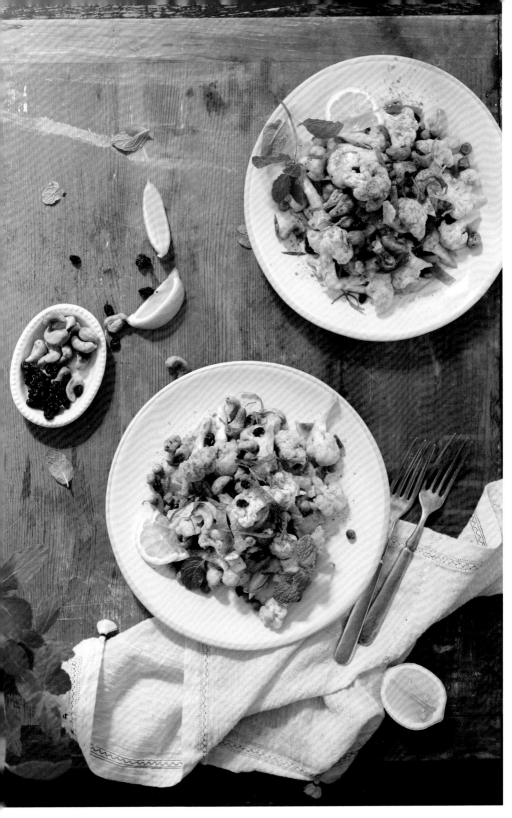

Curried Cauliflower with Peas and Mint (page 157)

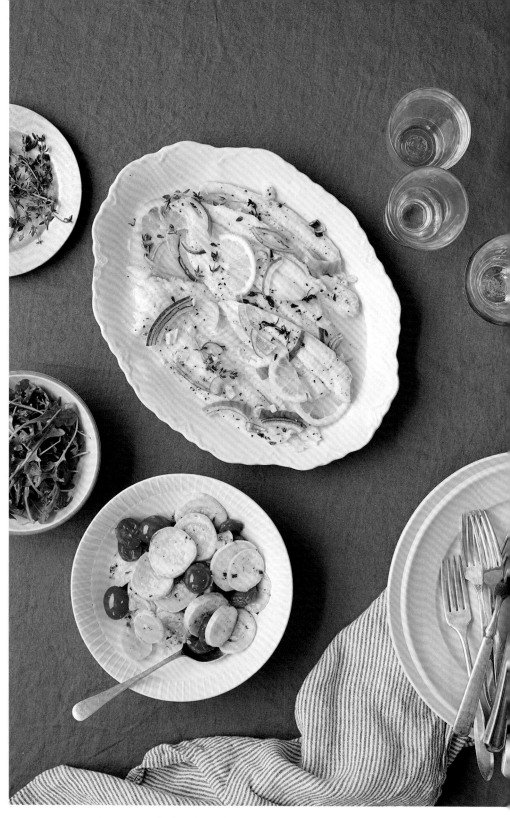

Lemon-Baked Sole with Stewed Summer Squash (page 176)

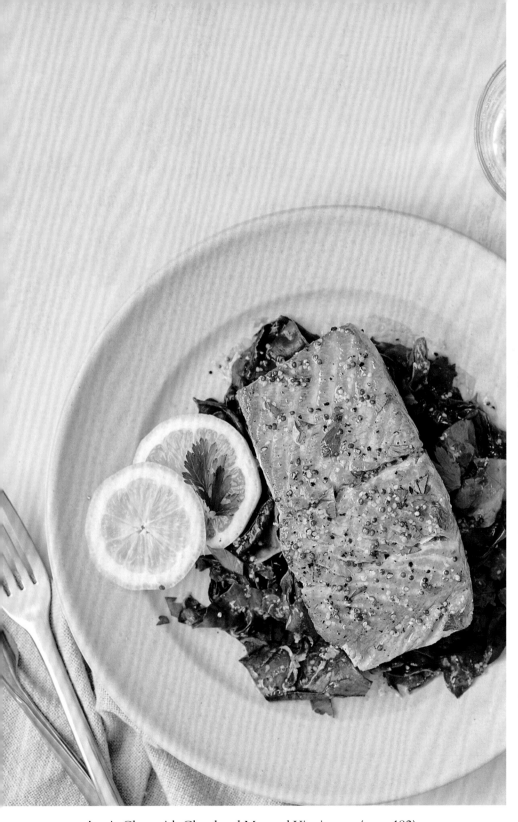

Arctic Char with Chard and Mustard Vinaigrette (page 182)

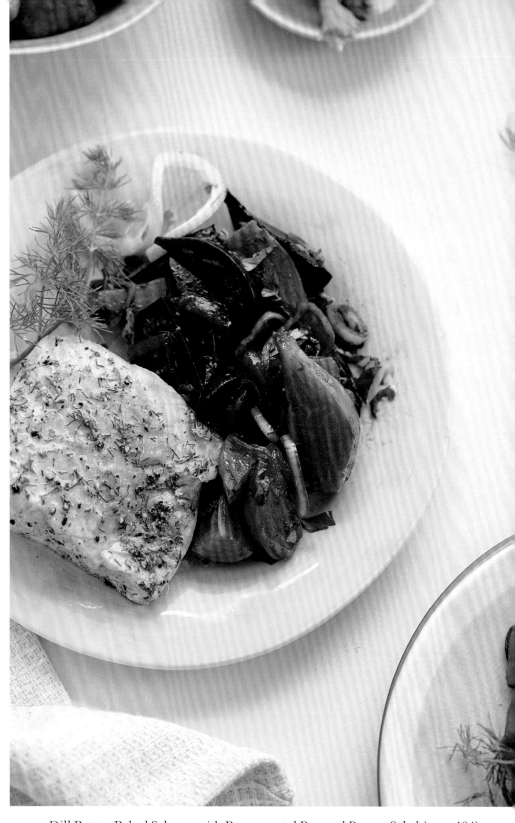

Dill Butter–Baked Salmon with Beetroot and Roasted Pepper Salad (page 184)

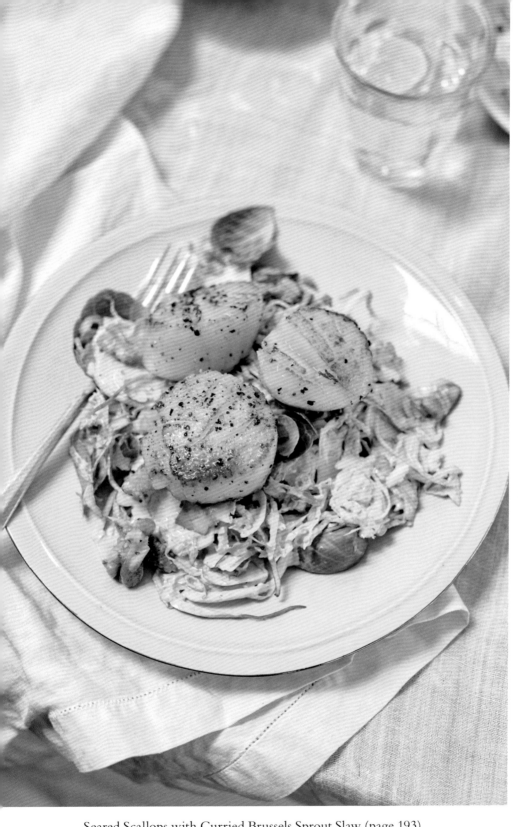

Seared Scallops with Curried Brussels Sprout Slaw (page 193)

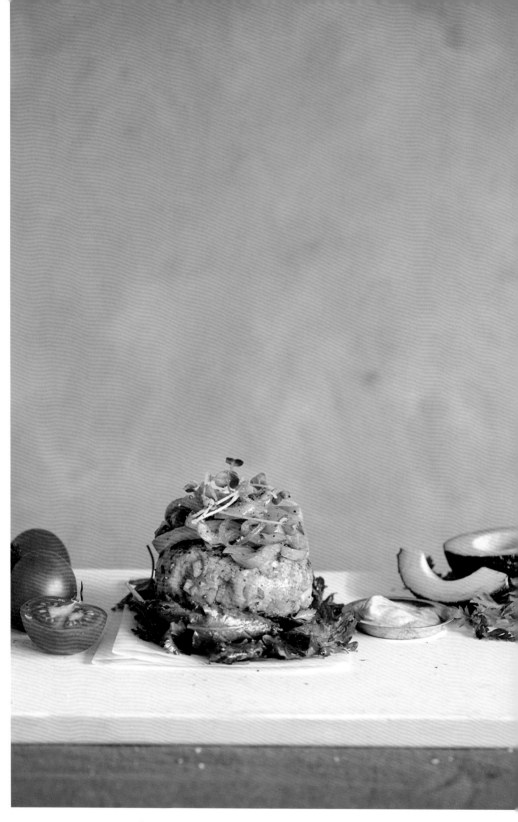

Turkey Burgers with Peppers and Onions (page 220)

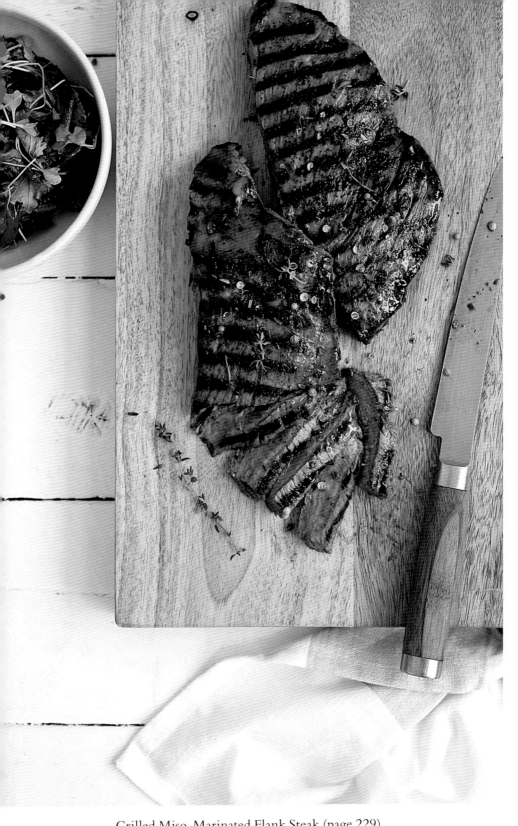

Grilled Miso–Marinated Flank Steak (page 229)

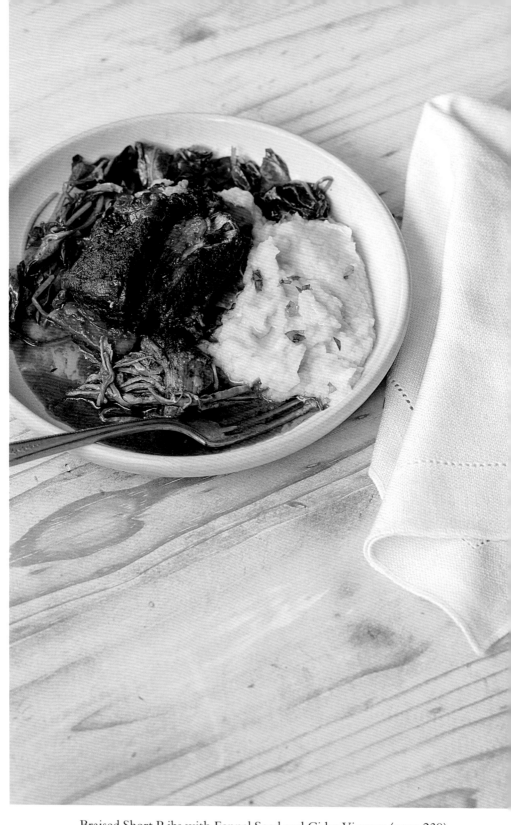

Braised Short Ribs with Fennel Seed and Cider Vinegar (page 239)

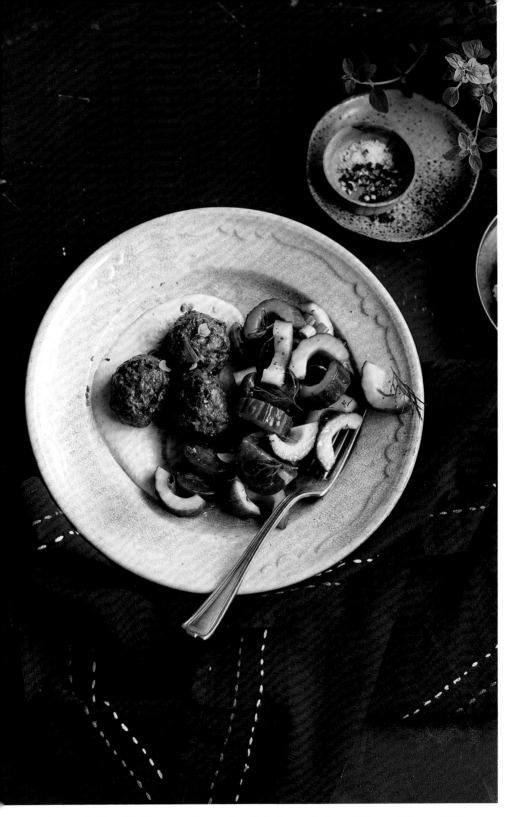

Lamb Meatballs with Tomato–Cucumber Salad and Cashew "Yogurt" (page 245)

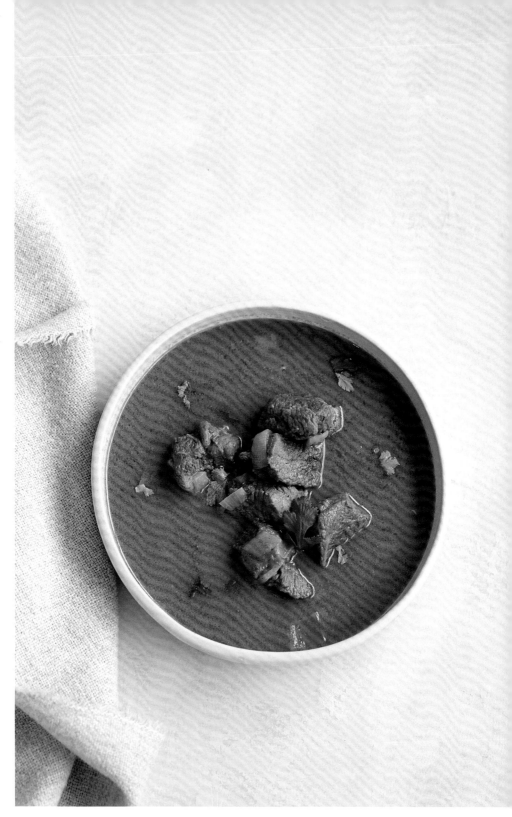

Caribbean Lamb Stew (page 247)

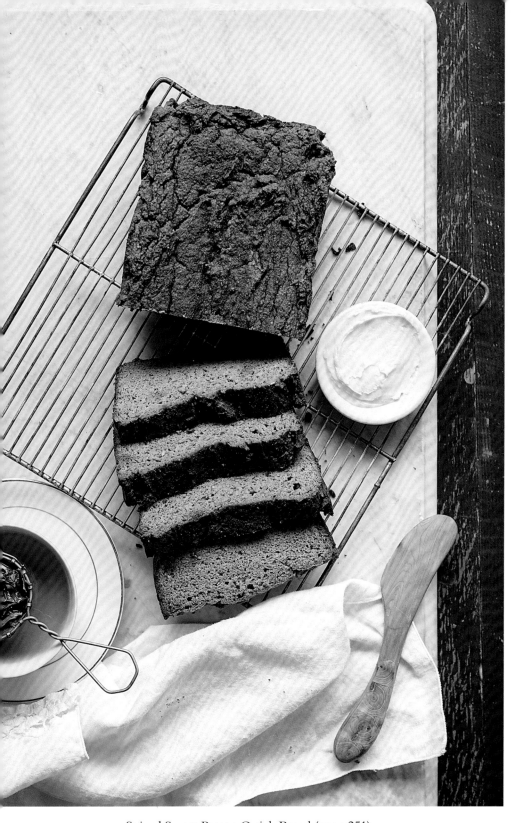

Spiced Sweet Potato Quick Bread (page 251)

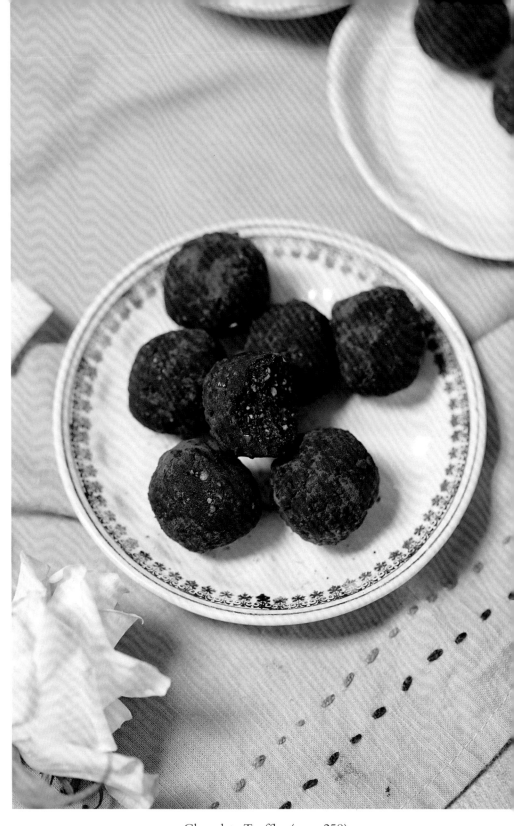

Chocolate Truffles (page 258)

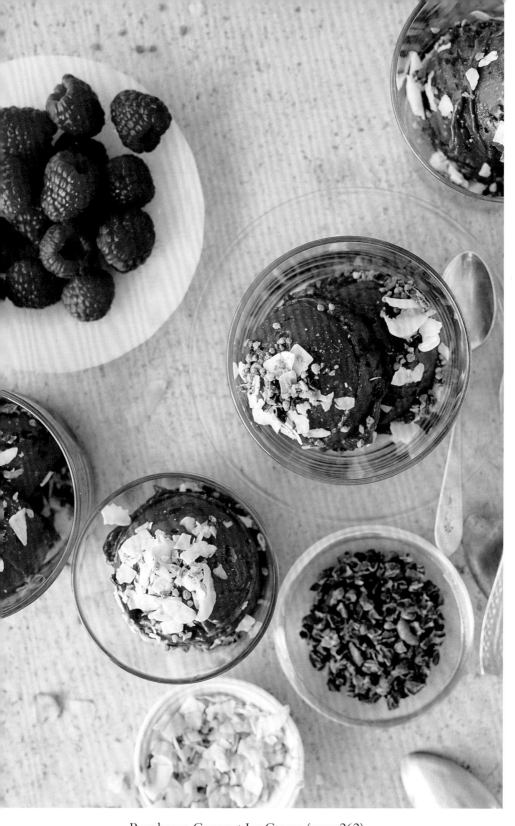

Raspberry–Coconut Ice Cream (page 262)

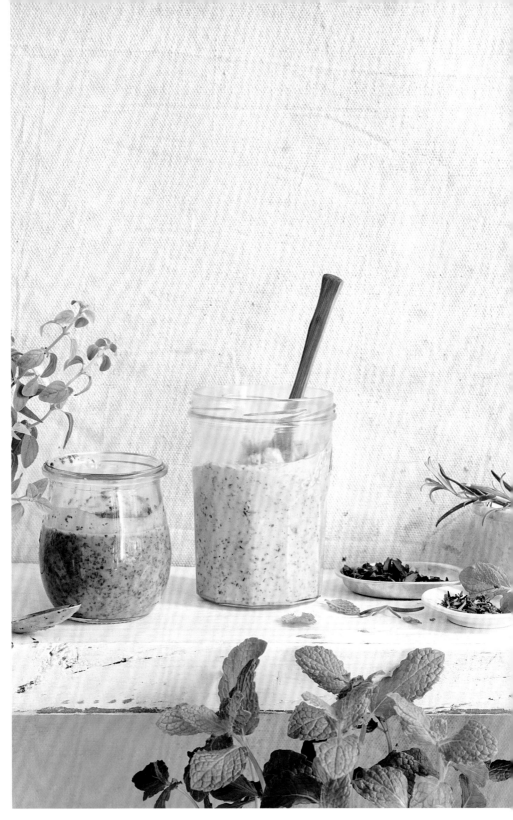

Chimichurri (page 272) and Herbed Compound Butter (page 280)

Use 1 tablespoon of the butter to grease a baking dish large enough to hold the salmon in a single layer. Place the fillets in it. Put the remaining butter in a small bowl, add the dill and the remaining ¼ teaspoon pepper and mix with a spoon until well combined. Spread the dill butter on the salmon fillets, dividing it equally. Squeeze the juice of half a lemon over each fillet. Bake the salmon until firm but the very center of the fillets is still translucent, 8 to 10 minutes.

Divide the salad between 4 plates. Place a salmon fillet on each plate and serve.

Nutritional analysis per serving: *Calories: 520, Fat: 43 g, Saturated Fat: 21 g, Cholesterol: 174 mg, Fiber: 3 g, Protein: 25 g, Carbohydrates: 10 g, Sodium: 776 mg*

SALMON WITH RED CABBAGE AND ORANGE SALAD

PEGAN DIET

A sweet-and-sour salad offsets the fattiness of wild salmon, my favorite fish. This dish is fresh-tasting and filled with vibrant colors, making it as pleasing for the eye as it is for the stomach. I prefer the flavor and texture of salmon when it's a little underdone in the center, but feel free to cook the fillets to your liking.

Serves: 4
Prep time: 15 minutes
Cook time: 10 minutes

- 4 x 100–125-g skin-on wild salmon fillets
- 4 tablespoons extra-virgin olive oil
- 1 teaspoon sea salt
- ¼ teaspoon freshly ground black pepper
- 2 oranges
- 1 small red cabbage, cored and shredded
- 50 g mint leaves, chopped
- 5 g basil leaves, chopped
- 2 tablespoons rice vinegar

Preheat the oven to 180°C/350°F/Gas 4.

Place the salmon in a baking dish large enough to hold the fillets in a single layer. Drizzle with 2 tablespoons of the olive oil, then sprinkle with ½ teaspoon of the salt and the pepper. Rub the oil and seasonings all over the fillets and bake until firm to the touch, 8 to 10 minutes.

While the fish bakes, cut the top and bottom off an orange. Stand it on a chopping board and use a sharp knife to cut away the rind and white pith in strips from top to bottom, following the contours of the fruit. Lay the orange on its side and cut it into round slices 5 mm thick. Repeat with the remaining orange.

Place the orange slices in a large bowl with the cabbage, mint, basil, vinegar, remaining 2 tablespoons oil and the remaining salt. Toss until well mixed.

Place a salmon fillet on 4 serving plates. Divide the salad between the plates and serve.

Nutritional analysis per serving: *Calories: 410, Fat: 25 g, Saturated Fat: 8 g, Cholesterol: 128 mg, Fiber: 5 g, Protein: 28 g, Carbohydrates: 21 g, Sodium: 704 mg*

Kimchi and Sweet Potato FishCakes with Cabbage-Apple Slaw

PEGAN DIET

Here spicy, garlicky kimchi is tempered by mashed sweet potatoes and mild-flavored white fish. You can prep the fishcakes the night before, then cook them and make the slaw just before you're ready to eat.

Serves: 4
Prep time: 30 minutes
Cook time: 10 minutes

- 1 small red cabbage, shredded
- 1 Granny Smith apple, cored and julienned
- 1 sweet red pepper, seeded and julienned
- 10 g fresh coriander leaves, roughly chopped
- 2 tablespoons fresh mint leaves, roughly chopped
- 2 tablespoons rice vinegar
- 2 tablespoons extra-virgin olive oil
- 1 teaspoon sea salt
- 750 g haddock fillets
- 225 g sweet potatoes, peeled and cut into 2.5-cm chunks
- 2 tablespoons unsalted, grass-fed butter
- 75 g drained kimchi, roughly chopped
- 2 spring onions, thinly sliced
- 1 large egg, beaten
- 3 tablespoons coconut flour
- coconut oil, for cooking
- 1 lime, cut into 8 wedges

Put the cabbage in a large bowl with the apple and pepper and toss to combine. Add the coriander, mint, vinegar, 1 tablespoon of the olive oil and ½ teaspoon of the salt. Mix until thoroughly combined. Cover and refrigerate until you're ready to serve.

Warm the remaining olive oil in a large frying pan over a medium-high heat until shimmering. Carefully add the fish and cook for 3 minutes, then flip them over. Cover, reduce the heat to medium, and continue to cook until the fillets are opaque and firm, 3 to 4 more minutes. Transfer the fish to a plate and allow to cool.

Place the sweet potatoes in a small saucepan and pour in 250 ml filtered water. Cover, bring to a simmer over a medium-high heat, and cook until the sweet potatoes are completely tender, about 8 minutes. Drain in a colander, then return them to the saucepan. Add the butter and, using a potato masher, smash them together, keeping mixture slightly chunky.

Transfer the sweet potatoes to a bowl and gently fold in the fish, kimchi, spring onions, egg and coconut flour. Stir in the remaining salt. Form the mixture into 8 equal patties about 5 cm in diameter and 2.5 cm thick.

Warm 2 tablespoons coconut oil in a large frying pan over a medium-high heat until shimmering. Carefully add the fishcakes and cook until lightly browned, about 3 minutes. Flip the fishcakes, adding more coconut oil if the pan is dry, and continue to cook until the underside of the cakes is lightly browned and they are heated through, about 3 more minutes.

Arrange 2 fishcakes on serving plates and mound the slaw alongside. Add 2 lime wedges to each plate and serve.

Nutritional analysis per serving: *Calories: 622, Fat: 31 g, Saturated Fat: 16 g, Cholesterol: 204 mg, Fiber: 9 g, Protein: 47 g, Carbohydrates: 28 g, Sodium: 917 mg*

Scampi Sauce

Prawns are great for heart health and nervous system support.

Serves: 4
Prep time: 15 minutes
Cook time: 15 minutes

- 4 tablespoons extra-virgin olive oil
- 450 g large prawns, peeled and deveined
- 1 large onion, thinly sliced
- 1 tablespoon crushed garlic
- 1 large tomato, roughly chopped
- 125 ml white wine
- 1 teaspoon sea salt
- ¼ teaspoon freshly ground black pepper
- 2 tablespoons unsalted, grass-fed butter
- 15 g fresh parsley leaves, roughly chopped

Warm 2 tablespoons of the olive oil in a large frying pan over a medium-high heat until shimmering. Add the prawns in an even layer and cook without stirring until lightly browned, about 1 minute. Flip each prawn and continue to cook until lightly browned on the underside, about 1 more minute; the prawns might not be fully cooked at this point, but that's okay. Transfer them to a plate and set aside.

Return the pan to a medium-high heat with the remaining olive oil. Add the onion and garlic and cook, stirring occasionally, until the onion begins to soften, about 3 minutes. Add the tomato, stir, then pour in the wine and simmer until slightly reduced. Add 65 ml filtered water and simmer until the sauce is reduced by half, about 8 minutes.

Add the prawns to the sauce, toss gently to coat, and cook until they are opaque throughout, 2 to 3 minutes. Season with the salt and pepper, stir in the butter and parsley, and serve.

Nutritional analysis per serving: *Calories: 326, Fat: 21 g, Saturated Fat: 6 g, Cholesterol: 236 mg, Fiber: 1 g, Protein: 25 g, Carbohydrates: 6 g, Sodium: 851 mg*

PRAWNS WITH SWEET POTATOES, KALE AND COCONUT MILK

This is a super-simple yet deeply nourishing one-pot recipe that combines good-quality fats from coconut milk, ghee and prawns with nutrient-dense veggies and healing spices.

Serves: 4
Prep time: 15 minutes
Cook time: 10 minutes

- 2 tablespoons Ghee (page 279)
- 2 large sweet potatoes, peeled and finely diced
- 2 tablespoons peeled and grated fresh ginger
- 2 teaspoons ground turmeric
- 250 ml full-fat coconut milk
- 450 g large prawns, peeled and deveined
- 100 g kale or cavolo nero, stemmed and roughly chopped
- 1 teaspoon sea salt
- 2 tablespoons fresh lime juice
- 10 g fresh coriander leaves

Warm the ghee in a 25-cm frying pan over a medium-high heat until shimmering. Add the sweet potatoes, toss to coat with the ghee, and cook until almost tender, 3 to 4 minutes. Stir in the ginger and turmeric, then pour in the coconut milk. Bring to a simmer, then add the prawns and scatter the kale on top. Cover and cook until the prawns are opaque throughout and the kale is wilted, about 3 minutes. Stir in the salt and lime juice.

Divide the prawns, vegetables and sauce equally between 4 bowls. Garnish with the coriander and serve.

Nutritional analysis per serving: *Calories: 486, Fat: 30 g, Saturated Fat: 23 g, Cholesterol: 221 mg, Fiber: 5 g, Protein: 29 g, Carbohydrates: 27 g, Sodium: 929 mg*

Scallops Meunière

In classic French cooking, *meunière* is a preparation of sautéed flour-dredged fish served with browned butter, lemon and parsley. This spin puts coconut flour on the scallops and includes lemon slices in the buttery sauce.

Serves: 4
Prep time: 15 minutes
Cook time: 10 minutes

- 50 g coconut flour
- 1 teaspoon sea salt
- ½ teaspoon freshly ground black pepper
- 12 large sea scallops (about 450 g), side muscles removed, patted dry
- 8 tablespoons unsalted, grass-fed butter
- 1 lemon, cut into 5-mm slices
- 10 g fresh parsley leaves, roughly chopped

Put the coconut flour in a bowl with the salt and pepper and whisk together. Taking 2 or 3 at a time, dredge the scallops in the seasoned flour, shake off the excess and place them on a plate.

Warm 2 tablespoons of the butter in a large frying pan over a medium-high heat until foaming. Add half the scallops and cook until golden brown, about 3 minutes. Flip them over and cook just until firm, about 1 more minute; do not overcook or they will become rubbery. Transfer the scallops to a platter and cover with foil to keep warm. Add 2 tablespoons of the remaining butter to the frying pan and cook the remaining scallops.

Wipe out the frying pan, set it over a medium–high heat, and add the remaining butter. Add the lemon slices and cook until they begin to soften, about 2 minutes. Stir in the parsley.

Pour the sauce (including the lemon slices) over the scallops and serve.

Nutritional analysis per serving: *Calories: 166, Fat: 3 g, Saturated Fat: 2 g, Cholesterol: 35 mg, Fiber: 5 g, Protein: 21 g, Carbohydrates: 12 g, Sodium: 854 mg*

SEARED SCALLOPS WITH CURRIED BRUSSELS SPROUT SLAW

This dish is elevated comfort food that's both easy to prepare and delicious.

Serves: 4
Prep time: 30 minutes
Cook time: 5 minutes

- 220 g Homemade Mayonnaise (page 265)
- 1 tablespoon curry powder
- 1 tablespoon apple cider vinegar
- ½ teaspoon freshly ground black pepper
- 450 g Brussels sprouts, trimmed
- 1 large carrot, scrubbed and grated
- 4 spring onions, green parts only, thinly sliced
- 60 g toasted walnuts, roughly chopped
- 1 teaspoon sea salt
- 12 large sea scallops (about 450 g), side muscles removed, patted dry
- 2 tablespoons Ghee (page 279)
- 1 lemon, cut into 4 wedges

Put the mayonnaise into a small bowl, add the curry powder, vinegar and ¼ teaspoon of the pepper and whisk together. Set aside.

Using a mandoline, or a food processor, or a sharp knife, slice the Brussels sprouts as finely as possible, then place in a large bowl. Add the carrot, spring onions, walnuts and mayonnaise mixture and stir until well combined. Season with ½ teaspoon of the salt, then set aside.

Season the scallops with the remaining salt and pepper. Warm the ghee in a large frying pan over a high heat until shimmering. Add the scallops to the pan in a single layer and cook until golden brown, about 3 minutes. Using tongs, carefully flip each scallop and cook for 1 more minute.

Place 3 scallops on each serving plate and spoon the slaw alongside. Serve with the lemon wedges.

Nutritional analysis per serving: *Calories: 456, Fat: 19 g, Saturated Fat: 5 g, Cholesterol: 0 mg, Fiber: 7 g, Protein: 34 g, Carbohydrates: 17 g, Sodium: 808 mg*

Coconut-Simmered Scallops with Quick-Pickled Vegetables

Creamy, with a little bit of heat and tartness, this quick-cooking dish packs a lot of flavor. The crisp, tangy "pickled" vegetables contrast pleasantly with the tender scallops and rich sauce. As the scallops are thinly sliced and begin to "cook" in the acidic marinade, take extra care not to overcook them on the hob.

Serves: 4
Prep time: 30 minutes
Cook time: 10 minutes

- 450 g large sea scallops, side muscles removed, cut in half across the grain
- 125 ml full-fat coconut milk
- 2 tablespoons fresh lime juice
- 4 teaspoons fish sauce
- 2 teaspoons ground coriander
- 1 small jalapeño chili, sliced into thin rounds
- 300 g sugarsnap peas, cut diagonally into thirds
- 1 large sweet red pepper, seeded and thinly sliced
- 1 large cucumber, trimmed and sliced into 5-mm rounds
- 2 tablespoons rice vinegar
- 1 tablespoon toasted sesame oil
- 1 tablespoon extra-virgin olive oil
- ½ teaspoon sea salt
- 70 g roughly chopped unsalted roasted cashews

Place the scallops in a non-metallic baking dish and add the coconut milk, lime juice, fish sauce, coriander and chili. Gently stir with a fork, then set aside to marinate while you prepare the vegetables.

Place the sugarsnaps, red pepper and cucumber in a large bowl. Add the vinegar, sesame oil, olive oil and salt and toss until well combined. Set aside for 20 to 30 minutes to "pickle".

Heat a medium frying pan over medium heat for 2 minutes, then pour in the scallops along with the marinade. Cook, stirring gently and occasionally, until the scallops are just opaque throughout, about 5 minutes; do not overcook.

Divide the scallops and sauce equally between 4 plates, then spoon the vegetables alongside. Sprinkle with the cashews and serve.

Nutritional analysis per serving: *Calories: 363, Fat: 24 g, Saturated Fat: 7 g, Cholesterol: 37 mg, Fiber: 2 g, Protein: 23 g, Carbohydrates: 17 g, Sodium: 706 mg*

Thai Red Curry with Seafood and Vegetables

I love Thai curry, but I resist ordering it in restaurants because of the sugar it contains. For that reason, I was determined to include a recipe in this book for Thai curry that's suitable for the *Eat Fat, Get Thin* Plan. My version is filled with all the requisite bold flavors, as well as with phytonutrients from the broccoli, peppers and coriander. It will not disappoint!

Serves: 4
Prep time: 20 minutes
Cook time: 25 minutes

- 2 tablespoons avocado oil
- 1 small onion, cut into large dice
- 1 large carrot, scrubbed and cut into 5-mm rounds
- 5-cm piece fresh ginger, peeled and grated
- 3 garlic cloves, crushed
- 2 tablespoons Thai red curry paste
- 1 x 400-ml can full-fat coconut milk
- 1 tablespoon fish sauce
- 1 large sweet red pepper, seeded and sliced into 5-mm strips
- 1 small head broccoli, stems peeled and cut into thin rounds, florets cut into bite-sized pieces
- 225 g large prawns, peeled, deveined and cut into thirds
- 225 g sea scallops, side muscles removed, cut horizontally into thin rounds
- 450 g mussels, scrubbed and debearded
- 25 g fresh coriander leaves, roughly chopped
- 1 lime, cut into 4 wedges

Warm the avocado oil in a 25-cm frying pan over a medium–high heat until shimmering. Add the onion and carrot and cook, stirring occasionally, until the onion begins to soften, about 2 minutes. Stir in the ginger and garlic and cook until fragrant, about 1 minute. Stir in the curry paste and cook for 1 minute, then pour in the coconut milk and add the fish sauce, stirring to combine. Bring to a simmer, then add the red pepper and broccoli. Reduce the heat to medium, cover and cook, stirring occasionally, until the broccoli is al dente, about 10 minutes. Add the prawns, scallops and mussels and stir to combine. Re-cover the pan and cook until the mussels open, about 5 minutes.

Discard any mussels that haven't opened. Ladle the curry into 4 bowls, garnish with the coriander, and serve with the lime wedges. You can also offer with Cauliflower "Rice" (page 156) if you wish.

Nutritional analysis per serving (without the Cauliflower Rice): *Calories: 503, Fat: 28 g, Saturated Fat: 17 g, Cholesterol: 107 mg, Fiber: 3 g, Protein: 37 g, Carbohydrates: 24 g, Sodium: 1128 mg*

Zuppa di Pesce

Here we have a classic Italian seafood stew with a tomato and wine base. It's essential to use really fresh fish and shellfish, as they will have the best flavor and be most nutritious. I prefer the stew made with a combination of wild-caught, firm-textured white fish, mussels, clams, prawns and squid, but the fundamental rule is to use the freshest and most appealing fish and seafood you can find.

Serves: 4
Prep time: 30 minutes
Cook time: 45 minutes

- 2 x 400-g cans whole peeled tomatoes
- 4 tablespoons extra-virgin olive oil.
- 1 large onion, roughly chopped
- 4 garlic cloves, crushed
- 15 g fresh parsley leaves, roughly chopped
- 1 teaspoon dried red chili flakes
- 250 ml dry white wine
- 750 g squid rings and/or large unshelled prawns
- 450 g skinless firm white fish fillets (such as snapper, cod, haddock, striped bass), cut into 2.5-cm chunks
- 450 g mussels and/or clams, scrubbed and debearded (if using mussels)
- sea salt
- ¼ teaspoon freshly ground black pepper

Place the tomatoes and their juice in a blender or food processor and purée until smooth.

Warm the olive oil in a large saucepan over a medium heat until shimmering. Add the onion and cook, stirring occasionally, until it begins to soften, 3 to 4 minutes. Stir in the garlic and half the parsley and cook until the garlic is fragrant, about 1 minute. Raise the heat to high, add the red chili flakes and wine and bring to a simmer. Continue simmering until the wine is reduced by half, about 3 minutes. Pour in the puréed tomatoes, bring back to a simmer and cook, stirring occasionally, for 5 minutes so that the flavors mingle.

Using a large spoon, begin adding the seafood to the pan in the following order: if using squid, add it first and cook for 10 minutes. Now add any prawns and white fish and cook for 2 minutes. Finally, add the mussels and/or clams, then reduce the heat to low and cook, uncovered, until the shellfish have opened, about 15 minutes. Season to taste with salt and stir in the black pepper.

Transfer the soup to a warmed tureen, discarding any mussels and/or clams that failed to open, and sprinkle with the remaining parsley. Bring the tureen to the table along with a ladle and serve in bowls.

Nutritional analysis per serving: Calories: 571, Fat: 22 g, Saturated Fat: 2 g, Cholesterol: 398 mg, Fiber: 2 g, Protein: 61 g, Carbohydrates: 21 g, Sodium: 177 mg

12

Poultry

SHREDDED CHICKEN

Making shredded or "pulled" chicken might seem like a lot of work, but it's easier than you might think. Gently simmering a whole chicken for 1½ hours breaks down the meat into tender pieces that flake off the bones with ease. Use the shredded meat in salads, toss it with Gingery Barbecue Sauce (page 277), or use it as a topping for Savory Coconut Pancakes (page 149).

Serves: 4
Prep time: 5 minutes
Cook time: 1½ hours, plus cooling

- 1 whole chicken (1.5–1.75 kg)
- 1 small onion, roughly chopped
- 3 garlic cloves, cut in half
- 1 tablespoon paprika
- 2 bay leaves
- 2 tablespoons apple cider vinegar

Place all the ingredients in a large saucepan or flameproof casserole dish and pour in 1 litre filtered water. Cover and bring to the boil over a high heat, then lower the heat and simmer until the chicken breaks apart easily and the meat is very tender, about 1½ hours.

Uncover the pan and set aside until the chicken is cool enough to handle. Lift it out, discard the cooking liquid and use your fingers to pick all the meat off the bones, shredding the large pieces. Discard the skin and bones. Use the shredded chicken right away, or refrigerate in an airtight container for up to 4 days.

Nutritional analysis per serving (200 g): *Calories: 589, Fat: 25 g, Saturated Fat: 9 g, Cholesterol: 315 mg, Fiber: 1 g, Protein: 81 g, Carbohydrates: 6 g, Sodium: 264 mg*

Chicken Escalopes with Mixed Greens

Escalopes are flattened pieces of meat and are extremely versatile. They can be served with a simple side dish, as they are here; they can be sliced and used as a component in a main-course salad; or they can even be topped with tomato sauce and baked. Chipotle Mayonnaise (page 267) is a delicious dipping sauce for chicken escalopes served on crisp lettuce.

Serves: 4
Prep time: 30 minutes
Cook time: 10 minutes

- 2 large boneless, skinless chicken breasts
- 30 g coconut flour
- 30 g teff flour
- 2 tablespoons potato flour
- ½ teaspoon sea salt, plus more for seasoning
- ½ teaspoon freshly ground black pepper
- 3 large eggs
- 2 tablespoons unsweetened Nut Milk (page 54)
- 60 g Ghee (page 279)
- 80 g mesclun
- 4 tablespoons extra-virgin olive oil
- 8 cherry tomatoes, cut in half
- 1 lemon, cut into 8 wedges

Place a chicken breast on a cutting board. Using a chef's knife, slice horizontally through the thickness of the breast, cutting it into 2 thin pieces. Repeat with the second chicken breast. Place the pieces one at a time between two sheets of clingfilm or baking parchment and gently pound with a meat mallet or heavy-based saucepan to an even thickness of 1 cm.

Put the coconut flour in a shallow baking dish with the teff flour, potato flour, ½ teaspoon salt and the pepper and stir together.

In a second shallow baking dish, whisk together the eggs and nut milk.

One at a time, dredge the escalopes in the flour mixture, shake off the excess, then dip into the egg mixture, coating both sides. Let the excess egg drip off, then dredge once again in the flour mixture. Set aside on a large plate.

Line a second large plate with kitchen paper. Warm the ghee in a large frying an over a medium–high heat until shimmering. Add the escalopes and cook until golden brown all over, 2 to 3 minutes per side. Transfer the escalopes to the paper-lined plate and season to taste with salt.

Divide the greens between 4 plates and drizzle each one with a tablespoon of the olive oil. Top each portion of greens with 4 cherry tomato halves and place a chicken escalope and 2 lemon wedges alongside. Serve.

Nutritional analysis per serving: *Calories: 474, Fat: 26 g, Saturated Fat: 7 g, Cholesterol: 237 mg, Fiber: 7 g, Protein: 35 g, Carbohydrates: 26 g, Sodium: 673 mg*

Sautéed Chicken and Vegetables

Even though we all live busy lives, we can still cook and eat nutritious, high-quality meals. With this chicken dish that's loaded with healthful veggies, you can get dinner on the table in less than 30 minutes *and* please everyone in the family.

Serves: 4
Prep time: 15 minutes
Cook time: 10 minutes

- 2 tablespoons Ghee (page 279)
- 2 large boneless, skinless chicken breasts, cut widthways into 1-cm strips
- 1 large red onion, thinly sliced
- 1 bunch asparagus, trimmed and cut widthways into quarters
- 2 large sweet red peppers, seeded and thinly sliced
- 200 g kale or cavolo nero, stemmed and roughly chopped
- juice of 1 lemon
- sea salt
- ½ teaspoon freshly ground black pepper

Warm the ghee in a large frying pan over a medium-high heat until it begins to smoke. Add the chicken strips and sauté until half-cooked, about 3 minutes. Add the onion, asparagus and red peppers and cook, stirring frequently, until the vegetables are tender, about 3 more minutes. Stir in the kale and lemon juice, then cover and cook, stirring occasionally, until the kale is wilted and tender, 2 to 3 minutes.

Season to taste with salt, stir in the black pepper, and serve.

Nutritional analysis per serving: *Calories: 263, Fat: 11 g, Saturated Fat: 5 g, Cholesterol: 86 mg, Fiber: 4 g, Protein: 29 g, Carbohydrates: 11 g, Sodium: 650 mg*

CHICKEN AND KELP NOODLE STIR-FRY

This recipe is great for using up leftover roasted or grilled chicken; slices of left-over steak work well too.

Serves: 4
Prep time: 20 minutes
Cook time: 10 minutes

- 2 tablespoons sesame oil
- 4 garlic cloves, crushed
- 2.5-cm piece fresh ginger, peeled and finely chopped
- 6 large white button mushrooms, thinly sliced
- 200 g shredded Chinese cabbage
- 1 sweet red pepper, thinly sliced
- 4 tablespoons coconut aminos
- 2 tablespoons rice vinegar
- 2 tablespoons Worcestershire sauce
- 225–275 g cooked boneless, skinless chicken breast, thinly sliced
- 450 g kelp noodles, cut into 5-cm lengths, soaked in warm water for 10 minutes, then drained
- 10 g coriander leaves, roughly chopped
- 4 spring onions, green parts only, thinly sliced
- 65 g roasted unsalted cashews, roughly chopped

Warm the sesame oil in a large frying pan over a high heat until shimmering. Add the garlic and ginger and cook, stirring constantly, until fragrant, about 1 minute. Add the mushrooms, toss a few times, then add the cabbage and red pepper. Cook, tossing frequently, until the vegetables have softened, 2 to 3 minutes. Pour in the coconut aminos, vinegar and Worcestershire sauce, stirring well after each addition. Add the chicken, stir to combine, and cook until just warmed through, 1 to 2 minutes. Add the kelp noodles and toss well. Stir in the coriander and spring onion greens. Divide the stir-fry between 4 plates, sprinkle with the cashews and serve.

Nutritional analysis per serving: *Calories: 287, Fat: 12 g, Saturated Fat: 2 g, Cholesterol: 508 mg, Fiber: 0 g, Protein: 14 g, Carbohydrates: 1 g, Sodium: 426 mg*

SLOW-COOKED CHICKEN WITH THAI FLAVORS

An amazingly tasty Thai-influenced chicken dish. Serve with Cauliflower "Rice" with Spring Onions (page 156).

Serves: 4
Prep time: 10 minutes
Cook time: 3 hours (unattended)

- 1 whole chicken (1.5–1.75 kg)
- 1 lime, thinly sliced
- 1 dried red chili
- 2.5-cm piece fresh ginger, peeled and finely chopped
- 5 garlic cloves, crushed
- 2 tablespoons finely chopped fresh lemongrass
- 2 teaspoons ground coriander
- 1 x 400-ml can full-fat coconut milk
- 2 tablespoons fish sauce
- ½ bunch coriander, stemmed and roughly chopped

Preheat the oven to 160°C/325°F/Gas 3.

Place the chicken in a large ovenproof casserole dish and add the lime slices, chili, ginger, garlic, lemongrass, coriander, coconut milk and fish sauce. Cover and cook in the oven for about 3 hours, occasionally basting with the cooking liquid, until the chicken is completely tender.

Carefully lift out the chicken and aside until cool enough to handle. At that point, pull the meat into large shreds and place in a bowl; discard the skin and bones. Spoon out and discard the lime left in the casserole dish, then pour the cooking liquid into a blender. Blend on high speed until well puréed, about 45 seconds. Pour the purée through a fine strainer set over the bowl containing the chicken. Stir the purée into the chicken until well combined. Sprinkle with the coriander and serve.

Nutritional analysis per serving: *Calories: 588, Fat: 58 g, Saturated Fat: 31 g, Cholesterol: 44 mg, Fiber: 4 g, Protein: 19 g, Carbohydrates: 34 g, Sodium: 887 mg*

CHICKEN CACCIATORE

The word *cacciatore* means 'hunters', and this rustic Italian dish is certainly rich enough to satisfy hearty appetites after a day's hunting in the woods or slaving at work. Although it can be on the table in just 60 minutes, the big, bold flavors make it tastes like it's been simmering for hours.

Serves: 4
Prep time: 10 minutes
Cook time: 1 hour

- 8 chicken drumsticks
- ½ teaspoon sea salt
- ½ teaspoon freshly ground black pepper
- 2 tablespoons Ghee (page 279)
- 1 small onion, thinly sliced
- 1 large carrot, scrubbed and finely diced
- 1 sweet red pepper, seeded and thinly sliced
- 3 garlic cloves, crushed
- 1 teaspoon finely chopped fresh rosemary
- 1 bay leaf
- 125 ml white wine
- 2 x 400-g cans whole peeled tomatoes, crushed by hand
- 100 g Kalamata olives, pitted and roughly chopped
- 2 tablespoons drained capers, roughly chopped
- 25 g fresh parsley leaves, roughly chopped

Season the drumsticks with the salt and pepper.

Warm the ghee in a 30-cm frying pan over a medium–high heat until shimmering. Add the drumsticks and cook, turning occasionally, until browned on all sides, 5 to 6 minutes in total. Transfer the chicken to a large plate, then add the onion, carrot and red pepper to the pan. Cook, stirring occasionally, until the vegetables are lightly browned, about 5 minutes. Stir in the garlic and rosemary, then add the bay leaf and wine. Using a wooden spoon, scrape up the browned bits on the bottom of the pan and simmer until the liquid has reduced by half, about 3 minutes. Stir in the tomatoes with their juice and return the drumsticks to the pan. Cover and simmer until the chicken is tender and opaque throughout, about 30 minutes.

Stir in the olives, capers and parsley. Place 2 drumsticks on each serving plate, generously spoon sauce over them and serve.

Nutritional analysis per serving: *Calories: 315, Fat: 15 g, Saturated Fat: 6 g, Cholesterol: 56 mg, Fiber: 5 g, Protein: 19 g, Carbohydrates: 21 g, Sodium: 792 mg*

Braised Chicken Thighs with Tomatillos

The dark meat on poultry thighs and drumsticks is rich and flavorful, but can be a bit tough, especially if it comes from good-quality free-range birds. Braising is a gentle cooking technique that tenderizes tough cuts, and it also results in a flavorful sauce to accompany the meat. Here cumin-seasoned chicken thighs are braised with tomatillos, onion and chili for a tasty dish with Mexican flair.

Serves: 4
Prep time: 15 minutes
Cook time: 45 minutes

- 8 boneless, skin-on chicken thighs
- 2 teaspoons ground cumin
- ¾ teaspoon sea salt
- ½ teaspoon freshly ground black pepper
- 1 tablespoon avocado oil
- 1 large onion, cut into 5-mm dice
- 3 garlic cloves, finely chopped
- 6 tomatillos, husked and quartered
- 1 jalapeño chili, thinly sliced
- 500 ml chicken stock
- 220 g Chipotle Mayonnaise (page 267)
- 5 g fresh coriander leaves, roughly chopped
- grated zest and juice of 1 lime
- 1 large avocado, stoned, peeled and cut into chunks

Season the chicken thighs with the cumin, salt, and pepper.

Warm the avocado oil in a flameproof casserole dish over a medium-high heat until shimmering. Place the chicken thighs in it, skin side down in a single layer, and cook until browned, 3 to 4 minutes. Flip the thighs and cook until the underside is lightly browned, about 2 minutes. Add the onion and garlic and cook, stirring occasionally, until the onion begins to soften, 1 to 2 minutes. Add the tomatillos, chili and chicken stock, and bring to the boil. Cover, and simmer until the chicken is tender and opaque throughout, about 30 minutes.

While the chicken cooks, put the chipotle mayonnaise in a small bowl and stir in the coriander, lime zest and juice.

Divide the chicken and sauce between 4 plates. Top each portion with a spoonful of the chipotle mayonnaise mixture and the avocado chunks and serve.

Nutritional analysis per serving: Calories: 627, Fat: 45 g, Saturated Fat: 10 g, Cholesterol: 164 mg, Fiber: 4 g, Protein: 39 g, Carbohydrates: 21 g, Sodium: 746 mg

Mustard-Orange Baked Chicken Legs with Wilted Radicchio

PEGAN DIET

Slightly bitter and spicy radicchio is a good source of antioxidants. Here it is paired with baked chicken to create a crowd-pleasing recipe. The combination of piquant mustard and bright, sweet orange adds bold flavor to the rich dark-meat parts of the chicken.

Serves: 4
Prep time: 15 minutes
Cook time: 45 minutes

- 4 skin-on chicken legs, divided at the joint into thighs and drumsticks
- 2 navel oranges, 1 juiced, 1 cut into 8 wedges
- 2 teaspoons paprika
- 1 teaspoon mustard powder
- 4 tablespoons extra-virgin olive oil
- 2 teaspoons red wine vinegar
- 2 teaspoons Dijon mustard
- 2 large heads radicchio, cored and shredded
- 1 tablespoon fresh lemon juice
- ½ teaspoon sea salt
- leaves from 3 thyme sprigs, finely chopped

Preheat the oven to 190°C/375°F/Gas 5.

Place the chicken pieces in a large bowl and add the orange juice and wedges, the paprika, mustard powder, half the olive oil, the vinegar and Dijon mustard. Toss until well combined and the chicken is evenly coated. Arrange the chicken pieces and orange wedges in a single layer in a baking tin. Bake for 30 minutes, then turn the chicken over and continue to bake until tender and opaque throughout, about 15 more minutes.

During the last 5 minutes of cooking time, warm the remaining 2 tablespoons olive oil in a large frying pan over a medium-high heat until shimmering. Add the radicchio and cook, stirring frequently, until completely wilted, about 3 minutes. Stir in the lemon juice and salt.

Scatter the radicchio on a platter, then arrange the chicken pieces and orange wedges on top. Sprinkle with the thyme and serve.

Nutritional analysis per serving: Calories: 453, Fat: 21 g, Saturated Fat: 4 g, Cholesterol: 122 mg, Fiber: 2 g, Protein: 24 g, Carbohydrates: 10 g, Sodium: 435 mg

CHICKEN, ASPARAGUS AND TOMATO WITH BROWN RICE

PEGAN DIET

After a long week of work or travel, I love to cook up a warm and comforting meal like this dish. It contains ingredients that provide deep nourishment, but if you're on the twenty-one-day *Eat Fat, Get Thin* Plan, substitute Cauliflower "Rice" (page 156) for the brown rice.

Serves: 4
Prep time: 15 minutes
Cook time: 20 minutes

- 160 g long-grain brown rice
- 550 ml chicken stock
- 2 tablespoons Ghee (page 279)
- 3 garlic cloves, crushed
- 2 large boneless, skinless chicken breasts, cut widthways into strips 1 cm thick
- 2 bunches asparagus, trimmed and cut into thirds
- 1 large tomato, roughly chopped
- 130 g tomato purée
- 250 ml chicken stock or filtered water
- leaves from 2 thyme sprigs, finely chopped
- ½ teaspoon sea salt
- ½ teaspoon freshly ground black pepper
- 2 tablespoons unsalted, grass-fed butter

Put the rice and chicken stock in a saucepan. Cover and bring to the boil over a high heat, then simmer until all the water is absorbed, about 15 minutes. Remove the pan from the heat and allow to stand, covered, for 5 minutes.

While the rice cooks, warm the ghee in a large frying pan over a medium-high heat until melted. Add the garlic and cook, stirring frequently, until it just starts to brown, about 2 minutes. Add the chicken, scattering the slices in a single layer, and cook without stirring; initially the slices will stick to the pan, but after about 3 minutes, when nearly half-cooked, they will release easily. At this point, add the asparagus, toss to combine, then add the tomato, tomato purée and chicken stock. Stir to combine, cover the pan and simmer until the chicken is cooked through and the asparagus is tender, about 3 minutes. Stir in the thyme, salt and pepper, then stir in the butter until incorporated.

Divide the rice between 4 bowls. Spoon the chicken mixture over the top and serve.

Nutritional analysis per serving: Calories: 422, Fat: 19 g, Saturated Fat: 10 g, Cholesterol: 106 mg, Fiber: 5 g, Protein: 36 g, Carbohydrates: 28 g, Sodium: 1781 mg

CHICKEN WITH SOFRITO AND SPINACH

Sofrito, a flavorful combination of slow-cooked, finely chopped aromatic vegetables, is a perfect seasoning for a mild-tasting chicken.

Serves: 4
Prep time: 15 minutes
Cook time: 1 hour

- 4 skin-on chicken legs
- 1 teaspoon sea salt
- 1 tablespoon Ghee (page 279) or lard
- 250 ml dry white wine
- 250 ml Dr. Hyman's Veggie-Bone Broth (page 128)
- 100 g Sofrito (page 284)
- 350 g baby spinach

Preheat the oven to 180°C/350°F/Gas 4.

Season the chicken legs with the salt. Warm the ghee in a large oven-proof frying pan over a medium-high heat until shimmering. Place the chicken skin side down in the pan and cook until browned, 4 to 5 minutes. Flip the legs and cook until the underside is lightly browned, about 2 minutes. Transfer to a large plate. Pour the wine into the pan and simmer until reduced by about half. Return the chicken legs, skin side up, to the pan. Pour in the bone broth, then place a quarter of the sofrito on top of each leg and use a spoon to spread it over the entire surface. Cover the pan, then place it in the oven and bake until the chicken is tender and opaque throughout, about 45 minutes.

Take the pan out of the oven and stir in the spinach. Re-cover and set aside to stand until the spinach is wilted, about 2 minutes.

Place a chicken leg on each serving plate, along with some of the spinach and sauce. Serve.

Nutritional analysis per serving: *Calories: 305, Fat: 17 g, Saturated Fat: 5 g, Cholesterol: 125 mg, Fiber: 3 g, Protein: 28 g, Carbohydrates: 9 g, Sodium: 748 mg*

Za'atar Roasted Chicken

Za'atar is the Arabic name for a thyme-like herb from the Middle East, but it is also the name for a seasoning blend based on the herb, which typically includes sesame seeds and sumac. It is often sprinkled onto flatbreads, but the flavors also work well with chicken. It can be bought in Middle Eastern food shops or online.

Serves: 4
Prep time: 5 minutes
Cook time: 1¼ hours

- 4 tablespoons salted, grass-fed butter
- 2 tablespoons za'atar
- 1 whole chicken (1.5–1.75 kg)
- 1 lemon, cut into 4 wedges

Preheat the oven to 220°C/425°F/Gas 7.

Warm the butter and za'atar in a small saucepan over a medium heat until the butter has melted.

Place the chicken in a baking dish and loosen the skin over the breasts. Brush some of the za'atar butter under the skin, directly onto the meat, then brush the remaining butter all over the exterior.

Roast the chicken for 20 minutes, then lower the temperature to 160°C/325°F/Gas 3 and continue to roast until the meat is opaque throughout and the thickest part of the breast registers 75°C/165°F on an instant-read thermometer, 40 to 45 more minutes.

Allow the chicken to rest for 5 minutes, then carve and serve with the lemon wedges.

Nutritional analysis per serving: *Calories: 677, Fat: 37 g, Saturated Fat: 16 g, Cholesterol: 346 mg, Fiber: 1 g, Protein: 81 g, Carbohydrates: 2 g, Sodium: 494 mg*

GRILLED CHICKEN BREASTS WITH SAMBAL

Sambal, a fiery chili paste, is a staple of Indonesian and Malaysian cuisine. Here a simple homemade sambal is used as a basting sauce for grilled chicken breasts. Sambal can also be used as a condiment, and it keeps in an airtight container in the refrigerator for a few days, so if you like spicy foods, I suggest making a double batch.

Serves: 4
Prep time: 20 minutes
Cook time: 30 minutes

- 1 tablespoon coconut oil
- 3 garlic cloves, thinly sliced
- 3 large spring onions, thinly sliced
- 10 fresh or dried Thai red chilies, stemmed, and seeded if you want less heat
- 1 large tomato, roughly chopped
- 1 tablespoon fish sauce
- grated zest and juice of 1 lime
- 4 x 175-g boneless, skin-on chicken breasts
- 2 tablespoons extra-virgin olive oil, plus extra for greasing
- ½ teaspoon sea salt

To make the sambal, warm the coconut oil in a 25-cm frying pan over a medium-high heat until melted. Add the garlic and spring onions and cook, stirring occasionally, until golden brown, 3 minutes. Add the chilies, tomato, fish sauce, lime zest and juice and cook, stirring occasionally, until the tomato begins to break down and its juice evaporates, about 10 minutes. Transfer the mixture to a blender and purée on high speed until smooth. Scoop the sambal into a small bowl and set aside. (It can be refrigerated in an airtight container for up to 5 days.)

Light a barbecue or preheat an oven grill to medium.

Coat the chicken breasts with the olive oil and season with the salt. Lightly grease the barbecue or grill rack with olive oil. Cook the chicken breasts skin side down until the skin is browned and releases easily from the rack, about 5 minutes. Flip the breasts, then use a pastry brush to spread sambal on each one. Continue to cook, basting once more with the remaining sambal, until the chicken is firm and opaque throughout, 3 to 4 more minutes. Transfer it, skin side up, to a cutting board and allow to rest for a few minutes.

Slice the chicken breasts against the grain and serve.

Nutritional analysis per serving: *Calories: 360, Fat: 22 g, Saturated Fat: 7 g, Cholesterol: 63 mg, Fiber: 2 g, Protein: 29 g, Carbohydrates: 12 g, Sodium: 725 mg*

Sautéed Chicken Hearts with Garlic and Rosemary

Often overlooked, chicken hearts are some of the most nutrient-dense parts of the bird, a great source of protein, B vitamins, zinc and iron. If you've never tried hearts, give this simple recipe a go. You'll be surprised by how delicious and satisfying they are.

Serves: 4
Prep time: 5 minutes
Cook time: 5 minutes

- 2 tablespoons Ghee (page 279)
- 4 large garlic cloves, thinly sliced
- 450 g chicken hearts, rinsed and patted dry
- 1 teaspoon finely chopped fresh rosemary
- ½ teaspoon sea salt
- ½ lemon

Warm the ghee in a large frying pan over a medium-high heat until shimmering. Add the garlic and cook, stirring occasionally, until lightly browned, about 2 minutes. Add the chicken hearts and cook, tossing continuously, until firm, about 4 minutes. Stir in the rosemary and salt, squeeze in the juice from the lemon half and serve.

Nutritional analysis per serving: *Calories: 248, Fat: 18 g, Saturated Fat: 8 g, Cholesterol: 154 mg, Fiber: 0 g, Protein: 18 g, Carbohydrates: 3 g, Sodium: 645 mg*

Turkey Burgers with Peppers and Onions

Turkey is a lean, neutral-flavored protein that pairs well with just about any type of seasoning. In this simple recipe, ground turkey meets curry powder, which boasts anti-inflammatory properties because of the spices it contains.

Serves: 4
Prep time: 15 minutes
Cook time: 20 minutes

- 450 g turkey mince
- 1 small onion, finely chopped, plus 1 large onion, thinly sliced
- 1 celery stick, finely chopped
- 2 tablespoons curry powder
- 1 large egg, beaten
- 1 tablespoon coconut flour
- 1 teaspoon sea salt
- 4 tablespoons coconut oil
- 2 sweet peppers, seeded and thinly sliced
- ½ teaspoon freshly ground black pepper
- 2 spring onions, thinly sliced
- 2 tablespoons chopped fresh parsley

Put the turkey meat in a bowl and add the chopped onion, celery, curry powder, egg, coconut flour and ½ teaspoon of the salt. Mix until thoroughly combined. Divide the mixture into 4 equal pieces and shape each into a 7.5-cm patty.

Warm 2 tablespoons of the coconut oil in a large nonstick frying pan over a medium heat until shimmering. Add the patties and cook until browned and firm and cooked through, about 7 minutes per side, flipping them just once.

Meanwhile, warm the remaining 2 tablespoons coconut oil in a large frying pan over a medium heat until shimmering. Add the sliced onion and peppers and cook, stirring occasionally, until softened, about 10 minutes. Stir in the remaining salt plus the pepper, spring onions and parsley.

Place a burger on each serving plate. Top with the onion and pepper mixture, dividing it evenly, and serve. This dish pairs nicely with a small bed of greens and avocado (optional).

Nutritional analysis per serving: *Calories: 417, Fat: 23 g, Saturated Fat: 10 g, Cholesterol: 152 mg, Fiber: 6 g, Protein: 36 g, Carbohydrates: 19 g, Sodium: 693 mg*

SLOW-COOKED DUCK LEGS WITH SPICED CHERRY SAUCE AND WHITE BEAN PURÉE

PEGAN DIET

Duck may be a bit pricey, but it's a great source of monounsaturated fat, so it's worth the indulgence. The deep, rich flavor of the meat pairs well with fruits and spices, and I particularly like the combination in this recipe. If you omit the white bean purée, you can enjoy this dish during the twenty-one-day plan.

Serves: 4
Prep time: 10 minutes
Cook time: 1¾ hours

- 4 duck legs
- ½ teaspoon sea salt
- ¼ teaspoon freshly ground black pepper
- 1 tablespoon Ghee (page 279)
- 150 g fresh or defrosted sweet cherries, stoned
- 1 litre Dr. Hyman's Veggie-Bone Broth (page 128)
- 2 whole star anise
- 5 cardamom pods
- 1 vanilla pod, cut in half lengthways
- 1 quantity White Bean Purée with Rosemary (page 150), warmed

Preheat the oven to 160°C/325°F/Gas 3.

Season the duck legs with the salt and pepper. Warm the ghee in a large flameproof casserole over a medium-high heat until melted. Place the duck legs in it skin side down and cook until lightly browned and some of the fat has rendered, 4 to 5 minutes. Pour off the fat, then add the cherries, bone broth, star anise, cardamom and vanilla pods. Bring to the boil, then cover and transfer the dish to the oven. Cook until the meat is tender and the cooking liquid is slightly reduced, about 1½ hours.

Transfer the duck legs to a plate and cover with foil to keep warm. Pour the cooking liquid through a fine-mesh sieve set over a small saucepan; discard the solids in the sieve. Set the pan over a low heat and bring the cooking liquid to a simmer.

Divide the bean purée between 4 plates and place a duck leg on top. Spoon a few tablespoons of the cooking liquid over each portion and serve.

Nutritional analysis per serving: *Calories: 306, Fat: 15 g, Saturated Fat: 5 g, Cholesterol: 105 mg, Fiber: 2 g, Protein: 27 g, Carbohydrates: 15 g, Sodium: 932 mg*

13

Beef and Lamb

MINCED BEEF AND BUTTERNUT SAUTÉ

I love the balance of sweet, spicy and herbal in this quick-cooking one-pot dish. Although the recipe calls for butternut squash, you can substitute any winter squash or root vegetable you prefer or have on hand.

Serves: 4
Prep time: 15 minutes
Cook time: 20 minutes

- 2 tablespoons Ghee (page 279)
- 1 large onion, finely diced
- 450 g grass-fed ground beef
- 2 teaspoons paprika
- ¾ teaspoon sea salt
- ½ small butternut squash, peeled, seeded and shredded (about 450 g)
- leaves from 2 x 10-cm rosemary sprigs, finely chopped

Warm the ghee in a large frying pan over a medium-high heat until melted. Add the onion and cook, stirring occasionally, until softened, 3 to 4 minutes. Add the beef and use a spatula to break it up and combine it with the onion. Cook until the meat is no longer pink, 3 to 4 minutes. Add the paprika and salt and cook, stirring occasionally, for 5 minutes. Add the shredded squash and continue to cook, stirring occasionally, until it is tender and the beef is thoroughly cooked, about 2 minutes. Stir in the rosemary.

Divide the mixture between 4 plates and serve.

Nutritional analysis per serving: *Calories: 320, Fat: 13 g, Saturated Fat: 6 g, Cholesterol: 60 mg, Fiber: 6 g, Protein: 25 g, Carbohydrates: 31 g, Sodium: 518 mg*

"Spaghetti" and Meatballs with Tomato Sauce

This is my kind of Sunday supper to enjoy with the family. Spaghetti squash baked until tender and separated into-noodle-like strands is a perfect gluten-free replacement for regular pasta. To help simplify cooking, the squash can be cooked the day before and reheated on the hob while the meatballs simmer in the sauce.

Serves: 4
Prep time: 15 minutes
Cook time: 30 minutes

- 2 tablespoons extra-virgin olive oil
- 1 large spaghetti squash, halved lengthways and seeded
- 450 g grass-fed minced beef
- 1 small onion, finely chopped
- 1 teaspoon garlic powder
- 30 g fresh parsley leaves, roughly chopped
- 1 teaspoon sea salt
- ½ teaspoon freshly ground black pepper
- 2 teaspoons fennel seeds, coarsely ground in a spice grinder
- 1 teaspoon dried red chili flakes
- 1½ tablespoons chia seeds, ground in a spice grinder
- 2 tablespoons unsalted, grass-fed butter, at room temperature
- 4 garlic cloves, thinly sliced
- 2 x 400-g cans fire-roasted tomatoes, roughly chopped (if unavailable, add a dash of liquid smoke to regular canned tomatoes, or add 200 g sun-blush tomatoes to 600 g canned tomatoes)

Preheat the oven to 180°C/350°F/Gas 4.

Drizzle 1 tablespoon of the olive oil over a baking sheet. Place the squash halves on it cut side down and bake until tender, about 25 minutes.

Meanwhile, put the beef into a bowl and add the onion, garlic powder, parsley, salt, black pepper, fennel seeds, red chili flakes and chia seeds. Mix until thoroughly combined. Using your hands, form the mixture into 12 equal meatballs and set aside.

When the squash is done, remove it from the oven, carefully flip over the squash halves and leave to stand until cool enough to handle.

Using a spoon, scrape the squash flesh from the skin, separating it into spaghetti-like strands. Transfer to a saucepan, add the butter and toss until well coated. Cover and keep warm on low heat until ready to serve.

Warm the remaining 1 tablespoon olive oil in a frying pan over a medium heat until shimmering. Add the sliced garlic and cook, stirring occasionally, until lightly browned, about 2 minutes. Stir in the tomatoes with their juice, then cover and cook for 5 minutes. Add the meatballs, re-cover the pan, and continue to simmer, stirring occasionally, until the meatballs are firm, about 20 minutes.

Divide the spaghetti squash between 4 plates. Top each portion with meatballs and several spoonfuls of sauce and serve.

Nutritional analysis per serving: *Calories: 768, Fat: 20 g, Saturated Fat: 7 g, Cholesterol: 75 mg, Fiber: 10 g, Protein:*

44 g, Carbohydrates: 115 g, Sodium: 963 mg

Meatloaf with Italian Seasonings

PEGAN DIET

Whenever I can, I spend a little extra time in the kitchen on Sundays to prepare for the week ahead. Dishes like meatloaf are fantastic because they can be cooked in advance and eaten over several days.

Serves: 4
Prep time: 15 minutes
Cook time: 30 minutes

- 50 g ground almonds
- 750 g grass-fed minced beef
- 1 large onion, finely chopped
- 30 g coconut flour
- 200 ml Smoky Ketchup (page 276)
- 3 large eggs, lightly beaten
- ½ bunch parsley, stemmed and roughly chopped
- 2 teaspoons dried thyme
- 1 teaspoon dried oregano
- ½ teaspoon freshly ground black pepper
- 1 tablespoon extra-virgin olive oil

Preheat the oven to 180°C/350°F/Gas 4.

Put the almond meal in a large bowl and add the beef, onion and coconut flour, 50 ml of the ketchup, the eggs, parsley, thyme, oregano and pepper. Mix until thoroughly combined, but do not overwork the mixture.

Drizzle the olive oil into the bottom of a 23 x 33-cm baking dish. Place the beef mixture in it and use your hands to form it into a 10 x 10-cm loaf about 5 cm high. Spread the remaining ketchup over the top.

Bake until the internal temperature of the meatloaf reaches 70°C/160°F on an instant-read thermometer, about 20 minutes. Remove the meatloaf from the oven and baste it. Cut into 2.5-cm slices and serve.

Nutritional analysis per serving: *Calories: 423, Fat: 21 g, Saturated Fat: 7 g, Cholesterol: 195 mg, Fiber: 14 g, Protein: 25 g, Carbohydrates: 34 g, Sodium: 617 mg*

Grilled Miso-Marinated Flank Steak

This marinade infuses the flavors of miso paste and dulse into a lean and usually tough cut of meat. Make sure to slice the steak against the grain so that it's as tender as can be. Enjoy this with Garlic-steamed Chard (page 159).

Serves: 4
Prep time: 10 minutes, plus marinating time
Cook time: 10 minutes

- 550 g beef flank steak
- 2 tablespoons chickpea miso
- 2 tablespoons dulse flakes
- 2 tablespoons wheat-free tamari
- 2 tablespoons toasted sesame oil
- 1 tablespoon rice vinegar
- 1 tablespoon coriander seeds, coarsely ground in a spice grinder
- 1 bunch spring onions, white parts only, thinly sliced
- 1 dried red chili, crushed
- 1 tablespoon grated ginger
- olive oil, for greasing the rack (if using a barbecue)
- thyme sprigs, for garnish (optional)

Place the flank steak in a non-metallic dish just large enough to hold it in a single layer.

Put the miso in a small bowl with the dulse flakes, tamari, sesame oil, vinegar, coriander seeds, spring onions, chili and ginger and whisk until combined. Pour the mixture over the flank steak, then turn it a few times to coat evenly with the marinade. Cover and refrigerate for 8 to 12 hours, turning the steak once.

Heat a barbecue until medium hot, then lightly grease the rack with olive oil. Alternatively, heat a large griddle pan over a medium-high heat. Remove the steak from the marinade and cook for 3 to 4 minutes per side for medium-rare (55°C/130°F); cook for less or more time, depending on your desired degree of doneness. Transfer the steak to a cutting board and leave to rest for 10 minutes.

Cut the steak against the grain into 1-cm slices and serve, garnished with the thyme, if using.

Nutritional analysis per serving: Calories: 379, Fat: 22 g, Saturated Fat: 6 g, Cholesterol: 94 mg, Fiber: 3 g, Protein: 34 g, Carbohydrates: 9 g, Sodium: 829 mg

GRILLED RED WINE AND ROSEMARY SIRLOIN STEAK WITH MUSHROOMS

I love the combination of beef, rosemary and mushrooms. Button mushrooms and portobellos are great, but to make the dish more interesting, try some unusual varieties such as oyster, chanterelle or black trumpet.

Serves: 4
Prep time: 15 minutes, plus marinating time
Cook time: 30 minutes

- 1 small shallot, thinly sliced
- 2 garlic cloves, crushed
- grated zest and juice of 1 lemon
- 125 ml red wine
- leaves from a 10-cm rosemary sprig, finely chopped
- ½ teaspoon sea salt
- ½ teaspoon freshly ground black pepper
- 2 x 225-g beef sirloin steaks
- 450 g mixed mushrooms (such as button, portobello, cremini, oyster and shiitake)
- 4 tablespoons extra-virgin olive oil, plus extra for greasing (if using a barbecue)
- 2 tablespoons fresh oregano leaves, roughly chopped
- leaves from 1 large thyme sprig, finely chopped

Place the shallot, garlic, lemon zest and juice in a non-metallic dish, add the wine, rosemary, salt and pepper and mix until the salt dissolves. Add the steaks and turn to coat with the marinade. Cover and refrigerate for 6 to 12 hours.

Heat a barbecue until medium-hot, then lightly grease the rack with olive oil. Alternatively, heat a large griddle pan over a medium-high heat. Meanwhile, trim any tough stems off the mushrooms and put the caps in a large bowl. Drizzle with 2 tablespoons of the olive oil, add the oregano and thyme, and toss to combine.

Remove the steaks from the dish, reserving the marinade, and barbecue or griddle for 3 to 4 minutes per side for medium-rare (55°C/130°F); cook for less or more time depending on your desired degree of doneness. A couple of minutes before the steaks are done, pour the reserved marinade over them and cook for 2 minutes so that the shallots and garlic flavor the meat. Transfer the steaks to a cutting board and leave to rest while you grill the mushrooms.

Carefully arrange the mushrooms on the barbecue rack or griddle pan and cook, turning them occasionally, until tender, about 5 minutes in total. Transfer the mushrooms to a platter, spreading them in an even layer.

Thinly slice the steaks on the diagonal and arrange the slices on the mushrooms. Drizzle with the remaining 2 tablespoons olive oil and serve.

Nutritional analysis per serving: Calories: 868, Fat: 37 g, Saturated Fat: 8 g, Cholesterol: 104 mg, Fiber: 68 g, Protein: 46 g, Carbohydrates: 109 g, Sodium: 395 mg

POT ROAST

Fork-tender pot roast and vegetables moistened with a herb-infused sauce is comfort food at its finest. Serve this dish with Cauliflower "Rice" with Spring Onions (page 156) or mashed sweet potatoes.

Serves: 4
Prep time: 10 minutes
Cook time: 3 to 4 hours (unattended)

- 1 x 900-g beef rump roasting joint
- 1 large onion, roughly chopped
- 4 large carrots, scrubbed and cut into big chunks
- 320 g cremini mushrooms, quartered
- 3 garlic cloves, crushed
- 525 g tomato purée
- 500 ml beef stock or filtered water
- 1 large bay leaf
- 2 thyme sprigs
- 1 teaspoon sea salt
- ½ teaspoon freshly ground black pepper

Preheat the oven to 160°C/325°F/Gas 3.

Place the beef in a large flameproof casserole dish, then add the remaining ingredients. Set the pan over a high heat and bring the liquid to the boil. Cover, transfer to the oven, and cook, basting the roast with the cooking liquid every 20 to 30 minutes, until the beef is fork-tender, 3 to 4 hours.

Transfer the roast to a chopping board and allow to rest for a few minutes. Cut the meat against the grain into 5-mm slices. Serve with the vegetables moistened with the cooking liquid.

Nutritional analysis per serving: *Calories: 486, Fat: 9 g, Saturated Fat: 2 g, Cholesterol: 128 mg, Fiber: 6 g, Protein: 63 g, Carbohydrates: 42 g, Sodium: 811 mg*

GINGERY BEEF AND VEGETABLE STEW WITH COCONUT MILK

In the winter, this stew is a staple for my family. It's easy to make, and so many of its ingredients are deeply nourishing.

Serves: 4
Prep time: 20 minutes
Cook time: 2½ hours (mostly unattended)

- 2 tablespoons Ghee (page 279)
- 2 large onions, roughly chopped
- 3 garlic cloves, crushed
- 2.5-cm piece fresh ginger, peeled and finely chopped
- 450 g stewing beef, in large chunks
- 2 large carrots, scrubbed and sliced into 5-mm rounds
- 250 ml Coconut Milk (page 55)
- 390 g tomato purée
- 450 g turnips, celeriac or swede, peeled and cut into 2.5-cm chunks
- 1 bunch kale, stemmed and roughly chopped
- ¾ teaspoon sea salt

Warm the ghee in a large flameproof casserole dish over a medium–high heat until shimmering. Add the onions and cook until softened and lightly browned, 3 to 4 minutes. Stir in the garlic and ginger, add the beef and cook until it begins to brown, 2 to 3 minutes. Add the carrots, coconut milk, tomato purée and 750 ml filtered water. Bring to the boil, then cover the dish, reduce the heat to medium–low, and simmer, stirring occasionally until the beef is tender, about 1½ hours.

Add the turnips, stir to combine, and continue to simmer until they are tender, about 25 minutes. Stir in the kale and salt and cook until the kale is wilted and tender, about 5 minutes.

Spoon the stew into bowls and serve.

Nutritional analysis per serving: *Calories: 479, Fat: 26 g, Saturated Fat: 15 g, Cholesterol: 75 mg, Fiber: 6 g, Protein: 28 g, Carbohydrates: 34 g, Sodium: 685 mg*

BALSAMIC BEEF STEW

This stew is an all-around healthy hit. The addition of balsamic vinegar adds a sweet and sour flavor that beautifully blends into the stew.

Serves: 4
Prep time: 5 minutes
Cook time: 2 hours

- 2 tablespoons Ghee (page 279)
- 1 large onion, roughly chopped
- 4 garlic cloves, crushed
- 2 tablespoons tomato purée
- 250 ml dry red wine
- 4 tablespoons balsamic vinegar
- 750 g stewing beef, in chunks
- 1 litre Dr. Hyman's Veggie-Bone Broth (page 128)
- 2 bay leaves
- 1 teaspoon dried thyme
- 2 carrots, scrubbed and cut into large chunks
- 3 celery sticks, diced
- 1 teaspoon sea salt

Warm the ghee in a large flameproof casserole dish over a medium heat until melted. Add the onion and cook, stirring occasionally, until softened and translucent, about 5 minutes. Stir in the garlic and cook until fragrant, about 1 minute. Add the tomato purée and cook until it darkens, stirring frequently, about 2 minutes. Pour in the wine and vinegar and simmer until reduced by about half. Add the beef, bone broth, bay leaves and thyme and stir to combine. Bring to a simmer, then cover partially and cook until the beef is tender, about 1½ hours.

Add the carrots and celery, stir to combine, and cook until the carrots are tender, about 30 minutes. Discard the bay leaves.

Stir in the salt. Spoon the stew into bowls and serve.

Nutritional analysis per serving: *Calories: 493, Fat: 27 g, Saturated Fat: 12 g, Cholesterol: 128 mg, Fiber: 2 g, Protein: 40 g, Carbohydrates: 15 g, Sodium: 618 mg*

Asian-Spiced Braised Beef with Baby Bok Choy

Tough cuts of meat, such as the silverside joint used here, do best with slow cooking, which helps to break down the muscle fibers and create a tender, yielding texture. Here I've paired it with baby bok choy, a vegetable with powerful antioxidants and anti-inflammatory properties.

Serves: 5
Prep time: 20 minutes
Cook time: 3 hours

- 1 tablespoon Ghee (page 279)
- 1 small onion, finely chopped
- 2.5-cm piece fresh ginger, peeled and finely chopped
- 1 x 1.5-kg beef silverside joint
- 2 teaspoons ground cloves
- 1½ teaspoons ground cumin
- 1½ teaspoons ground fennel seeds
- 5 whole star anise
- 4 bay leaves
- 3 cinnamon sticks
- 500 ml chicken stock
- 4 tablespoons low-sodium, wheat-free tamari
- 4 tablespoons mirin
- 4 heads baby bok choy, halved lengthways and cored
- 2 tablespoons toasted sesame seeds

Preheat the oven to 160°C/325°F/Gas 3.

Warm the ghee in a large flameproof casserole dish over a medium-high heat until melted. Add the onion and cook, stirring occasionally, until softened and translucent, 3 to 4 minutes. Stir in the ginger and cook until fragrant, about 1 minute. Add the beef and all the remaining ingredients, apart from the sesame seeds. Bring to the boil, cover the dish and cook in the oven for about 2½ hours, basting the beef every 20 to 30 minutes with the cooking liquid until it is fork-tender and easily breaks apart.

Transfer the beef to a cutting board, reserving the cooking liquid in the dish. Using two forks, pull the meat into large shreds.

Pour a 2.5-cm depth of water into a large saucepan and bring to the boil over a high heat. Place the bok choy in a steamer basket, set it over the pan, then cover and cook until tender, about 3 minutes.

Arrange the bok choy on a platter and top with the shredded beef. Pour the reserved cooking liquid through a fine-mesh sieve set over a bowl, then pour the liquid over the beef and bok choy. Sprinkle with the sesame seeds and serve.

Nutritional analysis per serving: *Calories: 730, Fat: 26 g, Saturated Fat: 10 g, Cholesterol: 197 mg, Fiber: 6 g, Protein: 84 g, Carbohydrates: 29 g, Sodium: 554 mg*

Slow-Cooker Beef Stew with Cabbage, Carrots and Mushrooms

The slow cooker is ideal for those of us who struggle to prepare healthful home-cooked dinners on weeknights. This recipe is perfect for it.

Serves: 4
Prep time: 20 minutes
Cook time: 8 to 10 hours (unattended)

- 1 large onion, roughly chopped
- 2 large carrots, scrubbed and cut into 5-mm rounds
- 3 celery sticks, cut into 1-cm pieces
- 275 g button mushrooms, quartered
- 1 green cabbage (900 g), cut into 8 wedges and cored
- 4 garlic cloves, thinly sliced
- 2 bay leaves
- 1 strip dried kelp (5 x 15 cm), snipped into small pieces
- 450 g stewing beef, in chunks
- 1 x 400-g can fire-roasted tomatoes, chopped (if unavailable, add a dash of liquid smoke to regular canned tomatoes, or add 200 g sun-blush tomatoes to 600 g canned tomatoes)
- 1 litre chicken stock
- ½ teaspoon freshly ground black pepper
- ½ bunch parsley, stemmed and roughly chopped
- 115 g unsalted, grass-fed butter, at room temperature

Put all the ingredients, apart from the parsley and butter, into a large slow cooker. Set the temperature to low and cook until the beef is fork–tender, 8 to 10 hours. Discard the bay leaves, then stir in the parsley. Spoon the stew into 4 bowls, dividing the beef and vegetables equally. Top each portion with 2 tablespoons of the butter and serve.

Nutritional analysis per serving: *Calories: 576, Fat: 39 g, Saturated Fat: 16 g, Cholesterol: 136 mg, Fiber: 8 g, Protein: 29 g, Carbohydrates: 31 g, Sodium: 640 mg*

Braised Short Ribs with Fennel Seed and Cider Vinegar

Short ribs are the perfect example of how a tough cut of meat can be transformed by cooking slow and low. A few hours in the oven and the ribs become fork-tender and succulent, and they absorb the flavors of the ingredients cooked with them. Bone broth as a braising liquid adds healing properties and lots of nutritional value to this rich and satisfying dish.

Serves: 4
Prep time: 5 minutes
Cook time: 2¾ hours (mostly unattended)

- 4 large beef short ribs, on the bone
- 3 garlic cloves, crushed
- 260 g tomato purée
- 500 ml Dr. Hyman's Veggie-Bone Broth (page 128)
- 1 tablespoon Dijon mustard
- 2 teaspoons ground fennel seeds
- 4 tablespoons apple cider vinegar
- ¾ teaspoon sea salt

Preheat the oven to 160°C/325°F/Gas 3.

Combine all the ingredients in a flameproof casserole dish and bring to the boil over a medium–high heat. Cover the dish, place it in the oven and cook until the meat is fork-tender, about 2½ hours.

Carefully transfer the short ribs to 4 shallow serving bowls. Using a spoon, skim off and discard as much fat as possible from the surface of the cooking liquid. Pour the liquid into a blender and blend on high speed until smooth, about 45 seconds. Pour the sauce over the short ribs, dividing it equally, and serve. This dish pairs nicely with cauliflower or sweet potato mash and a side of greens.

Nutritional analysis per serving: *Calories: 442, Fat: 37 g, Saturated Fat: 16 g, Cholesterol: 84 mg, Fiber: 2 g, Protein: 18 g, Carbohydrates: 7 g, Sodium: 608 mg*

Buffalo Burgers with Kelp Powder

Kelp, a natural detoxifier, is a wild ocean plant loaded with minerals. It has an earthy, savory flavor that works perfectly with the seasonings in these burgers. Buffalo meat is available online, but venison or grass-fed beef or lamb can be used instead.

Serves: 4
Prep time: 5 minutes
Cook time: 10 minutes

- 450 g minced buffalo meat
- 1 tablespoon onion powder
- 2 teaspoons paprika
- 2 teaspoons dried kelp powder
- 1½ teaspoons dried thyme
- 1 teaspoon dried oregano
- 1 teaspoon garlic powder
- 1 teaspoon sea salt
- olive oil, for greasing (if using a barbecue)

Place all the ingredients except the oil in a bowl and mix until thoroughly combined. Divide the mixture into 4 equal amounts and shape each into a 7.5-cm burger.

Heat a barbecue until medium hot, then lightly grease the rack with olive oil. Alternatively, heat a large griddle pan over a medium–high heat. Cook the burgers for 3 to 4 minutes per side for medium-rare (55°C/130°F); cook for less or more time depending on your desired degree of doneness. Serve.

Nutritional analysis per serving: *Calories: 269, Fat: 12 g, Saturated Fat: 4 g, Cholesterol: 50 mg, Fiber: 11 g, Protein: 23 g, Carbohydrates: 20 g, Sodium: 909 mg*

SHEPHERD'S PIE

In this recipe, mashed carrots and sweet potatoes stand in for the basic mashed potatoes that top a traditional shepherd's pie, giving this comfort-food classic a nutritional boost. The pie freezes nicely, so make it ahead and keep it on hand for those times when you're too busy to cook.

Serves: 6
Prep time: 30 minutes
Cook time: 45 minutes

- 450 g carrots, scrubbed and cut into 2.5-cm pieces
- 450 g sweet potatoes, peeled and cut into 2.5-cm chunks
- 1 tablespoon unsalted, grass-fed butter
- ½ teaspoon sea salt
- 1 tablespoon Ghee (page 279)
- 900 g minced lamb
- ½ large onion, finely chopped
- 2 teaspoons garlic powder
- 250 ml Dr. Hyman's Veggie-Bone Broth (page 128) or filtered water
- 2 tablespoons arrowroot
- 1 teaspoon finely chopped fresh rosemary

Put the carrots and sweet potatoes in a medium saucepan and pour in 500 ml filtered water. Cover, bring to the boil over a medium–high heat and cook until the vegetables are tender, about 8 minutes. Drain in a colander, then return them to the pan. Using a potato masher, mash the vegetables until smooth. Stir in the butter and salt. Cover to keep warm and set aside.

While the veg are cooking, warm the ghee in a large frying pan over a medium–high heat until melted. Add the lamb and cook, stirring occasionally, until it begins to brown, about 2 minutes. Add the onion and continue to cook, stirring occasionally, until it begins to soften, 3 to 4 minutes. Stir in the garlic powder, pour in the bone broth and bring to the boil. Lower the heat and simmer until the lamb is cooked through, about 5 minutes. Meanwhile, place the arrowroot in a small bowl and mix in 2 tablespoons filtered water. Stir this mixture into the lamb, increase the heat to medium-high and bring to the boil, stirring constantly, to thicken. Stir in the rosemary and remove from the heat.

Preheat the grill.

Pour the lamb mixture into a 23 x 33-cm flameproof baking dish, shaking the dish to form an even layer. Using a spatula, spread the carrot -sweet potato mash evenly over the lamb. Place under the grill until the pie is golden brown, 2 to 3 minutes.

Cut into squares and serve.

Nutritional analysis per serving: *Calories: 591, Fat: 41 g, Saturated Fat: 18 g, Cholesterol: 118 mg, Fiber: 5 g, Protein: 27 g, Carbohydrates: 28 g, Sodium: 381 mg*

GRILLED LAMB CHOPS WITH FRESH MINT AND BABA GHANOUSH

Baba ghanoush is a Middle Eastern aubergine purée flavored with tahini, lemon and olive oil. This version includes parsley, tomato and capers for added color and flavor. Although baba ghanoush is often served as a dip, here it's a wonderful side dish to grilled lamb chops.

Serves: 4
Prep time: 15 minutes
Cook time: 1 hour

- 2 large globe aubergines
- 3 garlic cloves
- ½ bunch parsley, stemmed
- 60 g tahini, plus more if needed
- 2 tablespoons fresh lemon juice, plus more if needed
- 1 teaspoon sea salt
- 1 small tomato, roughly chopped
- 2 teaspoons drained capers, finely chopped
- 8 lamb loin chops on the bone
- 4 tablespoons extra-virgin olive oil, plus extra for greasing (if using a barbecue)
- ½ teaspoon freshly ground black pepper
- 2 teaspoons thinly sliced fresh mint leaves

Preheat the oven to 190°C/375°F/Gas 5.

To make the baba ghanoush, poke the aubergines all over with a fork. Place them on a baking sheet and bake until softened and collapsed, 20 to 30 minutes. Set aside to cool completely.

Place a fine-mesh sieve over a bowl. Cut open the aubergines and spoon the flesh into the sieve; discard the skins. Leave to drain for 5 minutes, then transfer to a food processor. Add the garlic, parsley, tahini, lemon juice and ½ teaspoon of the salt. Pulse a few times to combine, then process until the mixture is smooth and creamy, about 1 minute.

Taste and add more tahini or lemon juice to suit your preference. Transfer the purée to a bowl, then fold in the tomato and capers. Cover and refrigerate until erquired.

Heat a barbecue until medium hot, then lightly grease the rack with olive oil. Alternatively, heat a grill until medium hot.

Drizzle the lamb chops with 2 tablespoons of the olive oil and season with the remaining salt and the pepper. Cook on the barbecue or under the grill for about 3 minutes per side for medium-rare (55°C/130°F); cook for less or more time depending on your desired degree of doneness.

Place 2 lamb chops on each serving plate and spoon baba ghanoush alongside them. Sprinkle each serving with 1 tablespoon of the mint leaves, drizzle with 1½ teaspoons of the remaining olive oil, and serve.

Nutritional analysis per serving: Calories: 418, Fat: 30 g, Saturated Fat: 7 g, Cholesterol: 0 mg, Fiber: 9 g, Protein: 20 g, Carbohydrates: 21 g, Sodium: 688 mg

LAMB MEATBALLS WITH TOMATO-CUCUMBER SALAD AND CASHEW "YOGURT"

With classic Middle Eastern flavors, these lamb meatballs make a great lunch or dinner. Make the cashew "yogurt" at least one day before you plan to serve the dish because it must stand at room temperature for several hours so that it ferments like real yogurt. After that, it can be chilled in the refrigerator.

Serves: 4
Prep time: 20 minutes, plus standing and chiling time
Cook time: 15 minutes

- 70 g raw cashews
- 1 tablespoon fresh lemon juice
- 2 tablespoons extra-virgin olive oil
- 450 g minced lamb
- 50 g fresh parsley leaves, roughly chopped
- 50 g fresh mint leaves, roughly chopped
- leaves from 2 large oregano sprigs, finely chopped
- 3 garlic cloves, crushed
- ¼ teaspoon dried red chili flakes
- 1 tablespoon chia seeds, ground in a spice grinder
- 275 g cherry tomatoes, cut in half
- 1 cucumber, peeled and sliced into 5-mm rounds
- 2 spring onions, thinly sliced
- 1 tablespoon apple cider vinegar
- sprinkle of fresh dill, for garnish (optional)

To make the cashew "yogurt," place the cashews, lemon juice and 6 tablespoons filtered water in a blender and blend on high speed until smooth and creamy, about 1 minute; add more water as needed to achieve a yogurt-like consistency. Pour the mixture into a glass container, cover and set aside at room temperature for 8 to 12 hours. Transfer to the refrigerator until cold, at least 1 hour or up to 3 days.

Preheat the oven to 180°C/350°F/Gas 4. Drizzle a 23 x 33-cm baking dish with 1 tablespoon of the olive oil.

To make the meatballs, put the lamb in a medium bowl and add the parsley, mint, oregano, garlic, red chili flakes and chia seeds. Mix well. Divide the mixture into 12 equal pieces and roll them into balls. Place in the prepared dish and bake until firm, 10 to 12 minutes.

To make the salad, put the tomatoes, cucumber and spring onions in a large bowl. Drizzle with the vinegar and the remaining tablespoon olive oil, and toss well.

Divide the salad between 4 plates, then place 3 meatballs alongside each serving. Drizzle generously with the cashew "yogurt", sprinkle on some fresh dill, if using, and serve.

Nutritional analysis per serving: Calories: 779, Fat: 68 g, Saturated Fat: 18 g, Cholesterol: 83 mg, Fiber: 4 g, Protein: 27 g, Carbohydrates: 20 g, Sodium: 89 mg

Caribbean Lamb Stew

When shopping, look for grass-fed lamb, one of the most nutritious animal proteins available because of the omega-3s and vitamin B_{12} it contains. The ginger, curry, coconut and especially the allspice give this stew a Caribbean flavor profile. Serve Cauliflower "Rice" with Spring Onions (page 156) on the side.

Serves: 4
Prep time: 10 minutes
Cook time: 2 hours

- 1 tablespoon coconut oil
- 450 g stewing lamb, in chunks
- 1 large onion, chopped
- 2.5-cm piece fresh ginger, peeled and finely chopped
- 1 tablespoon curry powder
- ½ teaspoon ground allspice
- 550 g tomato purée
- 1 x 400-ml can full-fat coconut milk
- 250 ml Dr. Hyman's Veggie-Bone Broth (page 128)
- ½ teaspoon sea salt
- sprinkle of parsley, for garnish (optional)

Warm the coconut oil in a large saucepan over a medium–high heat until shimmering. Add the lamb and cook, stirring occasionally, until lightly browned on all sides, 3 to 4 minutes. Add the onion and cook, stirring occasionally, until it begins to soften, about 2 minutes. Stir in the ginger, curry and allspice, then pour in the tomato purée, coconut milk and bone broth. Bring to the boil, then lower the heat, partially cover and simmer, stirring occasionally, until the lamb is fork-tender, about 2 hours. Stir in the salt.

Divide the stew between 4 serving bowls, sprinkle with the parsley, if using, and serve.

Nutritional analysis per serving: *Calories: 657, Fat: 36 g, Saturated Fat: 23 g, Cholesterol: 151 mg, Fiber: 9 g, Protein: 52 g, Carbohydrates: 38 g, Sodium: 401 mg*

Braised Lamb Shanks with Moroccan Flavors

Bring out those spices and put them to good use in this lamb dish inspired by Moroccan flavors. Not only do spices add flavor and fragrance to your meals; they also contain phytochemicals that can strengthen your immune system. So why not add a little spice to your life?

Serves: 4
Prep time: 10 minutes
Cook time: 4 hours (mostly unattended)

- 2 tablespoons Ghee (page 279)
- 1 large onion, finely chopped
- 3 large garlic cloves, crushed
- 2 teaspoons paprika
- 1½ teaspoons ground cumin
- 1 teaspoon ground coriander
- pinch of saffron threads
- 4 x 225-g lamb shanks
- 1 preserved lemon, thinly sliced
- 4 large carrots, scrubbed and quartered widthways
- ½ bunch coriander, stemmed and roughly chopped
- ½ teaspoon sea salt
- ½ teaspoon freshly ground black pepper

Warm the ghee in a flameproof casserole dish over a medium heat until shimmering. Add the onion and cook, stirring occasionally, until softened and translucent, about 5 minutes. Stir in the garlic and cook until fragrant, about 1 minute, then stir in the paprika, cumin, coriander and saffron and cook until the spices are fragrant, about 2 minutes. Place the lamb shanks in a single layer on top of the onion mixture. Pour in enough filtered water to come halfway up the shanks. Bring to the boil, then partially cover and simmer, basting and turning the shanks about every 30 minutes, until they are tender, about 3 hours.

Stir in the preserved lemon slices and carrots. Cover the dish again and cook, basting the shanks about every 15 minutes, until the carrots are tender, about 30 minutes. Stir in the coriander, salt and pepper.

Place the shanks in 4 shallow bowls, arrange the carrots and lemons alongside, and spoon sauce over each portion. Serve.

Nutritional analysis per serving: *Calories: 576, Fat: 27 g, Saturated Fat: 11 g, Cholesterol: 202 mg, Fiber: 1 g, Protein: 66 g, Carbohydrates: 13 g, Sodium: 695 mg*

14

Breads and Desserts

SPICED SWEET POTATO QUICK BREAD

Easy to make and naturally sweet from the sweet potatoes, this quick bread is perfect whenever you need a bread fix. It's especially good slathered with softened ghee or butter.

Makes: 1 loaf
Prep time: 10 minutes
Cook time: 1 hour

- 2 tablespoons coconut oil
- 2 large sweet potatoes, peeled and thinly sliced
- 55g coconut flour
- 1 tablespoon ground cinnamon
- 1 teaspoon ground nutmeg
- ½ teaspoon ground mace
- 1 teaspoon bicarbonate of soda
- 1 teaspoon baking powder
- generous pinch of sea salt
- 4 large eggs
- 125 g almond butter
- 4 tablespoons unsalted, grass-fed butter, melted
- 1 teaspoon organic almond extract

Preheat the oven to 180°C/350°F/Gas 4. Grease a 23 x 13-cm loaf tin with the coconut oil. Cut a piece of baking parchment to fit in the bottom of the tin and lay it inside.

Place the sweet potato slices in a medium saucepan and add enough filtered water to cover by 2.5 cm. Bring to the boil over a high heat and cook until tender, about 5 minutes. Drain in a colander, then return the potato slices to the saucepan. Using a masher, mash them until smooth, then set aside to cool to room temperature.

Put the coconut flour in a bowl with the cinnamon, nutmeg, mace, bicarbonate of soda, baking powder and salt.

Whisk the eggs in a separate large bowl until combined. Add the mashed sweet potatoes and the almond butter, melted butter and almond extract and whisk gently until well combined. Add the coconut flour mixture and mix with a rubber spatula until evenly incorporated. Pour the batter into the prepared tin and bake until a cocktail stick inserted into the center comes out clean, 50 to 60 minutes.

Turn the bread onto a wire rack and allow to cool completely. Cut the loaf into 2.5-cm slices and serve. It will keep at room temperature for up to 4 days if tightly wrapped in clingfilm.

Nutritional analysis per serving (1 slice): Calories: 405, Fat: 19 g, Saturated Fat: 7 g, Cholesterol: 95 mg, Fiber: 43 g, Protein: 9 g, Carbohydrates: 70 g, Sodium: 323 mg

Injera (Ethiopian Flatbread)

PEGAN DIET

Injera is a traditional food of Ethiopia. This soft, spongy bread is made with gluten-free teff flour, and fermentation gives it a tangy flavor. Serve the rounds of bread with any meal, use them as a base for your morning eggs, or simply spread them with butter and enjoy.

Makes: about 8
Prep time: 5 minutes, plus 1 to 2 days for fermentation
Cook time: 10 minutes

- 375 g teff flour
- 2 teaspoons sea salt
- 4 tablespoons Ghee (page 279) or extra-virgin olive oil, for cooking

Place the teff flour and salt in a bowl, pour in 1 litre filtered water and whisk to combine. The mixture should resemble loose pancake batter. Cover the bowl with a clean tea towel and set aside to stand at room temperature until small bubbles form in the batter, 1 to 2 days.

Warm 1½ teaspoons of the ghee in a 20-cm heavy-based frying pan over a medium heat until shimmering. Spoon about 4 tablespoons of the batter into a ladle, noting how high up it comes, then pour it into the center of the pan. Use a spatula to spread it into a 15-cm circle, and cook until completely dry on the surface, 4 to 5 minutes. Transfer the injera to a large plate and cover to keep warm. Cook the remaining batter in the same way, using additional ghee and stacking the injeras on the same plate.

Serve at room temperature. Interleave any leftovers with kitchen paper and refrigerate in a large ziplock bag for up to 4 days.

Nutritional analysis per serving (1 bread): *Calories: 237, Fat: 9 g, Saturated Fat: 5 g, Cholesterol: 15 mg, Fiber: 6 g, Protein: 6 g, Carbohydrates: 33 g, Sodium: 568 mg*

Lemon-Cashew "Curd" with Fresh Blueberries

PEGAN DIET

When wild blueberries ripen in the late summer, I always look forward to picking and eating the tiny fruits. The berries are loaded with antioxidants and deliver a pleasant balance of sweet and tart flavors. This lemony, blueberry-garnished cashew "curd" comes together easily in a blender and is a light, refreshing dessert.

Serves: 4
Prep time: 20 minutes, plus soaking and chiling time

- 275 g raw cashews
- 125 ml unsweetened cashew milk or filtered water
- 4 tablespoons fresh lemon juice
- grated zest of 2 lemons
- ½ teaspoon vanilla powder
- 1 tablespoon maple syrup
- 150 g blueberries
- 4 tablespoons bee pollen granules

Put the cashews in a medium bowl and cover with 1 litre filtered water. Set aside to soak at room temperature for 30 minutes.

Drain the cashews and rinse well. Transfer to a blender and add the cashew milk, lemon juice and zest, vanilla powder and maple syrup. Blend on high speed until the mixture is very smooth and creamy, about 1 minute.

Divide the "curd" between 4 wineglasses or dessert bowls. Cover and refrigerate until chilled, at least 2 hours or up to 8 hours.

Top each portion of chilled "curd" with a quarter of the blueberries, sprinkle with a tablespoon of the bee pollen and serve.

Nutritional analysis per serving: *Calories: 431, Fat: 30 g, Saturated Fat: 6 g, Cholesterol: 0 mg, Fiber: 6 g, Protein: 15 g, Carbohydrates: 35 g, Sodium: 3 mg, Sugars: 9 g*

PANNA COTTA WITH BLUEBERRIES AND PECANS

Panna cotta is a traditional Italian dessert with a custard-like texture. Its name translates to "cooked cream", but this version uses coconut milk. Blueberries and pecans hide at the bottom of each ramekin for a delicious surprise.

Serves: 4
Prep time: 30 minutes, plus cooling time
Cook time: 10 minutes

- 115 g blueberries, defrosted if frozen
- 30 g toasted pecans, roughly chopped
- 2 x 400-ml cans full-fat coconut milk
- 2 tablespoons unflavored powdered gelatine
- 1 teaspoon ground cinnamon
- ½ teaspoon vanilla powder

If using defrosted blueberries, drain them in a fine-mesh sieve to remove any excess moisture.

Place the blueberries and pecans in a small bowl and stir together. Divide equally between 4 ramekins.

Pour the coconut milk into a medium saucepan. Sprinkle the gelatine over the surface and leave to swell, about 5 minutes. Warm the mixture over a low heat, whisking constantly, just until the gelatine dissolves. Take off the heat and stir in the cinnamon and vanilla powder. Pour the mixture into the ramekins, dividing it equally, then cover and refrigerate until set, at least 4 hours or up to 8 hours.

Serve the chilled panna cotta in the ramekins.

Nutritional analysis per serving: *Calories: 291, Fat: 26 g, Saturated Fat: 18 g, Cholesterol: 0 mg, Fiber: 2 g, Protein: 6 g, Carbohydrates: 10 g, Sodium: 43 mg*

Chocolate-Avocado Pudding with Cinnamon

PEGAN DIET

Rich and creamy avocado is transformed into a simple no-cook pudding that will satisfy any chocolate lover's craving.

Serves: 4
Prep time: 30 minutes, plus chiling time

- 250 ml unsweetened Nut Milk (page 54)
- 4 Medjool dates, pitted
- 2 avocados, stoned and peeled
- 30 g cacao powder
- 1 teaspoon pure vanilla extract
- 1 teaspoon ground cinnamon
- generous pinch of sea salt
- 125 g raspberries

Warm the nut milk in a small saucepan over a low heat until just shy of simmering. Add the dates, remove the pan from the heat, and set aside to cool to room temperature. (You can speed up the cooling process by transferring the nut milk and dates to a bowl and refrigerating.)

Scoop the softened dates out of the nut milk and place them in a food processor, reserving the milk. Pulse the dates until broken up, about 6 pulses. Scrape down the sides of the bowl, add the avocados, and pulse until they are mostly smashed, 4 or 5 pulses. Add the cacao powder, vanilla, cinnamon, salt and reserved nut milk and process until the mixture is smooth and creamy.

Divide the pudding between 4 ramekins or dessert bowls. Cover and refrigerate until chilled, at least 1 hour or up to 8 hours.

Top the puddings equally with the raspberries and serve.

Nutritional analysis per serving: *Calories: 395, Fat: 13 g, Saturated Fat: 2 g, Cholesterol: 0 mg, Fiber: 40 g, Protein: 6 g, Carbohydrates: 82 g, Sodium: 129 mg, Sugars: 20 g*

CHOCOLATE-PISTACHIO FUDGE

PEGAN DIET

This easy recipe includes coconut milk, pistachios and cardamom to create a fudge with exotic flavors that you don't have to feel guilty about eating.

Makes: 12 pieces
Prep time: 15 minutes, plus chiling time

- 350 g dark chocolate, at least 70% cocoa solids, finely chopped
- 1 teaspoon vanilla powder
- ½ teaspoon ground cardamom
- ¼ teaspoon sea salt
- 1 tablespoon Ghee (page 279)
- 250 ml full-fat coconut milk
- 2 tablespoons maple sugar
- 30 g shelled raw pistachios, roughly chopped
- cacao powder, for dusting

Place the chopped chocolate in a large heatproof bowl and add the vanilla, cardamom and salt.

Put the ghee in a small saucepan with the coconut milk and maple sugar and warm over a medium-low heat, stirring to dissolve the sugar. When just shy of simmering, immediately pour the mixture over the chocolate. Stir until completely melted and the mixture is smooth and very thick. Gently stir in the pistachios.

Transfer the mixture to a lined prepared baking sheet and use a spatula to form it into a 15 x 20-cm slab about 1 cm thick. Refrigerate until the fudge is firm, at least 12 hours, or freeze for about 4 hours.

Cut the chilled slab into 12 squares, dust with cacao powder and serve. Store in an airtight container in the refrigerator for up to 7 days.

Nutritional analysis per serving (1 piece): *Calories: 115, Fat: 7 g, Saturated Fat: 4 g, Cholesterol: 508 mg, Fiber: 0 g, Protein: 14 g, Carbohydrates: 1 g, Sodium: 426 mg, Sugars: 6 g*

Chocolate Truffles

PEGAN DIET

Sweetened with dates, these little confections will satisfy when the craving strikes for something rich and chocolaty.

Makes: 20 truffles
Prep time: 20 minutes, plus chiling time

- 7 to 9 Medjool dates, pitted
- 140 g raw cashews
- 3 tablespoons cacao powder, plus extra for for dusting
- 1 teaspoon alcohol- and gluten-free pure vanilla extract
- 1 teaspoon ground nutmeg
- generous pinch of sea salt

Place 7 of the dates in a food processor, add the cashews, the measured amount of cacao powder, and the vanilla, nutmeg and salt. Process until the mixture is finely ground and begins to stick together, 45 to 60 seconds. Pinch off a marble-size piece and squeeze it in your hand to check it sticks together. If it doesn't, return it to the food processor, add the remaining 2 dates and process until well combined.

Transfer the mixture to a bowl. Using a small ice cream scoop or two spoons, form the mixture into 20 equal mounds and place on a small baking sheet. Roll 1 mound at a time into a firmly packed ball and place it back on the baking sheet.

Put about 2 tablespoons of cacao powder in a small bowl. Roll each truffle in it until coated on all sides, then return it to the baking sheet. Cover and refrigerate the truffles until firm, at least 1 hour or up to 1 week. Serve chilled.

Nutritional analysis per serving (1 truffle): *Calories: 588, Fat: 58 g, Saturated Fat: 31 g, Cholesterol: 0 mg, Fiber: 3 g, Protein: 3 g, Carbohydrates: 12 g, Sodium: 60 mg, Sugars: 8 g*

No-Bake Walnut Brownies

PEGAN DIET

Everybody loves a good brownie, but most are full of refined sugar and wheat flour. I've created a simple, no-bake version made with walnuts, which contain generous amounts of essential vitamins and minerals.

Makes: 8 brownies
Prep time: 15 minutes, plus chiling time

- 400 g raw walnuts
- 120 g cacao nibs
- 2 tablespoons cacao powder
- 2 Medjool dates, pitted
- 2 tablespoons unsalted, grass-fed butter, at room temperature
- 3 tablespoons melted cacao butter
- pinch of sea salt

Line the bottom of a 23-cm square baking dish with baking parchment.

Place all the ingredients in a food processor and process until the mixture is well combined and free of large chunks (it will be grainy), about 45 seconds.

Transfer the mixture to the prepared baking dish and, using your hands, press it into an even, firmly packed layer. Cover and refrigerate until firm, at least 2 hours or up to 4 days. The brownies can also be frozen for up to 3 months.

Cut the chilled brownies into 5-cm pieces and serve.

Nutritional analysis per serving (1 brownie): *Calories: 560, Fat: 48 g, Saturated Fat: 5 g, Cholesterol: 8 mg, Fiber: 4 g, Protein: 24 g, Carbohydrates: 18 g, Sodium: 28 mg, Sugars: 4 g*

Buckwheat and Apple Crepes with Cashew Cream

PEGAN DIET

Buckwheat flour has a nutty flavor that pairs perfectly with the maple sugar and cashew cream in this recipe. The crepes are best hot, so serve straight from the pan.

Serves: 4
Prep time: 5 minutes, plus resting time for the batter
Cook time: 15 minutes

- 240 g buckwheat flour
- 2 tablespoons maple sugar
- 1 teaspoon ground cinnamon
- ½ teaspoon ground ginger
- grated zest of 1 lemon
- ¼ teaspoon sea salt
- 2 large eggs, beaten
- 125 ml unsweetened Almond Milk (page 54)
- 4 tablespoons unsalted, grass-fed butter, melted and cooled, plus extra for frying
- 75 g cashews
- ¼ teaspoon vanilla powder
- 2 large crisp, tart apples

To make the crepe batter, put the buckwheat flour in a bowl, add the maple sugar, cinnamon, ground ginger, lemon zest and salt and whisk together. Whisk in the eggs and almond milk, then fold in the melted butter. Cover and set aside at room temperature for up to 1 hour, or refrigerate for up to 2 days.

To make the nut cream, put the cashews in a blender along with the vanilla powder and 125 ml filtered water. Blend on high for about 45 seconds, until creamy and free of lumps, adding more water if needed, until the cream is quite thick but runny. Transfer it to a screwtop jar and store in the fridge until required.

When you're ready to cook the crepes, peel, core and slice the apples into thin wedges.

Melt 1 tablespoon butter in a 20-cm frying pan over a medium heat. Measure 4 tablespoons of the batter into a ladle, noting how high it comes. Pour it into the center of the frying pan and use a spatula to spread it into a 10-cm circle about 5 mm thick. Carefully arrange a quarter of the apple slices in a pinwheel shape on the batter and cook until the crepe is lightly browned underneath, about 2 minutes. Using a metal spatula, carefully flip the crepe and cook until done, 2 to 3 minutes, adding more butter as needed to prevent sticking. Slide the crepe onto a plate with the apples facing up, top with cashew cream and serve.

Make 3 more crepes in the same way, and serve as before.

Nutritional analysis per serving (1 crepe?): *Calories: 503, Fat: 18 g, Saturated Fat: 9 g, Cholesterol: 123 mg, Fiber: 13 g, Protein: 14 g, Carbohydrates: 80 g, Sodium: 219 mg, Sugars: 17 g*

Raspberry-Coconut Ice Cream

Ice cream made with frozen fruit and coconut cream is every bit as rich and delicious as dairy-based ice cream. Here I use raspberries, which are a fantastic source of vitamin C and fiber. You don't need an ice-cream machine for this recipe, but for best results, use a high-speed blender that comes with a pusher so the berries purée thoroughly and the mixture is quick to turn smooth and creamy. The ice cream doesn't keep well, so be prepared to serve all of it immediately after blending.

Serves: 4
Prep time: 5 minutes

- 550 g frozen raspberries
- 150 g coconut cream
- 1 teaspoon alcohol- and gluten-free pure vanilla extract
- ½ teaspoon ground cardamom
- 2 tablespoons dark maple syrup (optional, for Pegan Diet)
- 2 tablespoons bee pollen granules
- 2 tablespoons shredded unsweetened coconut
- 2 tablespoons cacao nibs

Place the raspberries in a blender and add the coconut cream, vanilla, cardamom and maple syrup, if using. Blend on high speed, using the pusher (if available) to push the berries down towards the blade, until the mixture is smooth, thick, and creamy, about 1 minute.

Using a spatula, scoop the ice cream into 4 bowls. Sprinkle each portion with 1½ teaspoons each of the bee pollen, coconut shreds and cacao nibs and serve.

Nutritional analysis per serving: *Calories: 173, Fat: 3 g, Saturated Fat: 2 g, Cholesterol: 0 mg, Fiber: 12 g, Protein: 4 g, Carbohydrates: 26 g, Sodium: 8 mg, Sugars: 8 g*

PEACH ICE CREAM

PEGAN DIET

The combination of peaches and cream is a classic, but here coconut cream stands in for the dairy. As with the Raspberry-Coconut Ice Cream (page 262), you don't need an ice-cream machine to make this dessert, but a high-speed blender works best to create a smooth, creamy consistency.

Serves: 4
Prep time: 10 minutes

- 1 kg frozen peach slices
- 150 g coconut cream
- 65 ml coconut oil, softened
- 1 teaspoon vanilla powder
- 1 teaspoon ground mace
- 30 g cacao nibs, to serve

Place half the ingredients, apart from the cacao nibs, in a blender and blend on high speed, using the pusher (if available) to push the peaches down towards the blade, until the mixture is smooth, thick and creamy, about 1 minute. Transfer the mixture to a bowl and place it in the freezer. Prepare the remaining ingredients, apart from the cacao nibs, in the same way, and mix into the batch already in the freezer.

Scoop the ice cream into 4 bowls. Sprinkle each portion with 1 table-spoon of the cacao nibs and serve.

Nutritional analysis per serving: *Calories: 256, Fat: 25 g, Saturated Fat: 2 g, Cholesterol: 0 mg, Fiber: 4 g, Protein: 3 g, Carbohydrates: 19 g, Sodium: 5 mg*

15

Sauces, Condiments, and Seasonings

Homemade Mayonnaise

Once you taste homemade mayonnaise, you'll want to toss out the shop-bought stuff in your refrigerator. You can make it by hand for a great arm workout, or use a blender if you prefer.

Makes: 220 g
Prep time: 25 minutes

- 2 large egg yolks
- 1 tablespoon fresh lemon juice, plus extra as needed
- 1 tablespoon white wine vinegar or champagne vinegar
- ¼ teaspoon Dijon mustard
- 1 teaspoon sea salt
- freshly ground white pepper
- 250 ml avocado oil or extra-virgin olive oil

To make the mayonnaise by hand, place the egg yolks in a medium bowl with the lemon juice, vinegar, mustard, salt and a pinch of white pepper. Stabilize the bowl by resting it on bunched-up damp kitchen paper, then whisk the ingredients until well combined. While whisking continuously and vigorously, add the oil a few drops at a time. Once the mixture starts to thicken, add the remaining oil in a very slow, thin stream while continuing to whisk. If you add too much oil too quickly, the mixture will not thicken, so it's better to go slow. If necessary, you can stop for a moment to rest your arm or switch hands. After all the oil has been added, taste the mayonnaise and adjust the seasoning with pepper and/or lemon juice.

To make the mayonnaise in a blender, place the egg yolks in a small bowl with the lemon juice, vinegar, mustard, salt and a pinch of white pepper. Whisk until well combined. Transfer the mixture to a blender and blend on low speed for a few seconds. With the machine running, add the oil just a few drops at a time. Once the mixture starts to thicken, add the remaining oil in a very slow, thin stream. After all the oil has been added, taste the mayonnaise and adjust the seasoning with pepper and/or lemon juice.

Transfer the mayonnaise to a non-metallic container. Use right away or cover tightly and refrigerate for up to 4 days. If the mayonnaise gets too thick, whisk in up to 2 teaspoons cold filtered water to thin it.

Nutritional analysis per serving (1 tablespoon): *Calories: 100, Fat: 11 g, Saturated Fat: 2 g, Cholesterol: 25 mg, Fiber: 0 g, Protein: 0 g, Carbohydrates: 0 g, Sodium: 10 mg*

CHIPOTLE MAYONNAISE

You don't have to use the same old spreads and dips on this plan. Try this smoky chipotle mayonnaise for a change—you'll want to spread it on everything!

Makes: 220 g
Prep time: 10 minutes

- 125 ml sunflower oil
- 4 tablespoons extra-virgin olive oil
- 2 large egg yolks
- 1 tablespoon Dijon mustard
- 1 tablespoon fresh lemon juice
- ½ teaspoon chipotle powder
- 1 teaspoon sea salt

Combine the two oils in a measuring jug.

Place the egg yolks in a blender with the mustard, lemon juice, chipotle powder and salt and whiz for a few seconds to blend. With the machine running on low speed, add the oil just a few drops at a time. Once the mixture starts to thicken, add the remaining oil in a very slow, thin stream.

Transfer the mayonnaise to a non-metallic container. Use right away or cover tightly and refrigerate for up to 4 days. If the mayonnaise gets too thick, whisk in up to 3 tablespoons cold filtered water to thin it.

Nutritional analysis per serving (1 tablespoon): *Calories: 92, Fat: 9.5 g, Saturated Fat: 1.5 g, Cholesterol: 23 mg, Fiber: 0.5 g, Protein: 1.25 g, Carbohydrates: 1 g, Sodium: 150 mg*

Green Olive Tapenade

Tapenade is a savory spread made from olives, a staple ingredient in the Mediterranean store cupboard. The big, bold flavors of tapenade pair well with fish, chicken, lamb and roasted vegetables.

Makes: 325 g
Prep time: 15 minutes

- 300 g green olives, pitted
- 3 garlic cloves, roughly chopped
- 40 g hemp seeds
- 8 olive oil-packed anchovies, drained
- grated zest of 1 lemon
- juice of ½ lemon
- 1 teaspoon chopped fresh rosemary
- 30 g fresh parsley leaves, roughly chopped
- 4 tablespoons extra-virgin olive oil

Put the olives in a food processor with the garlic, hemp seeds, anchovies, lemon zest and juice, rosemary and parsley and pulse until the olives are roughly chopped, 4 or 5 pulses. With the machine running, add the olive oil in a steady stream and process until a coarse paste forms, about 1 minute. Scrape down the bowl and pulse a few more times to ensure that the mixture is well combined.

Transfer the tapenade to a bowl and serve, or store in an airtight container in the refrigerator for up to 1 week.

Nutritional analysis per serving (2 tablespoons): *Calories: 90, Fat: 7 g, Saturated Fat: 0 g, Cholesterol: 0 mg, Fiber: 1 g, Protein: 3 g, Carbohydrates: 13 g, Sodium: 99 mg*

ROCKET PESTO

Sometimes it's nice to shake things up a bit, as in this recipe, which swaps the usual sweet basil for peppery rocket. Nutritional yeast adds a cheesy flavor but keeps the recipe dairy-free.

Makes: 350 g
Prep time: 15 minutes

- 75 g baby rocket
- 45 g pine nuts
- 2 garlic cloves
- 60 ml extra-virgin olive oil
- 10 g nutritional yeast
- ½ teaspoon sea salt

Put the rocket, pine nuts and garlic in a food processor and pulse until the mixture is finely chopped, 4 or 5 pulses. Scrape down the sides of the bowl, then add the olive oil, nutritional yeast and salt. Process until well incorporated, about 30 seconds.

Use the pesto right away or refrigerate in an airtight container for up to 1 week. For longer storage, freeze the pesto in ice-cube trays until solid, then transfer to a ziplock bag and store in the freezer for up to 3 months.

***Nutritional analysis per serving (60 g):** Calories: 293, Fat: 31 g, Saturated Fat: 4 g, Cholesterol: 0 mg, Fiber: 1 g, Protein: 3 g, Carbohydrates: 3 g, Sodium: 151 mg*

Pecan Romesco

Romesco is a Spanish sauce made with nuts, tomato, garlic and peppers or chilies. This version uses pecans instead of the traditional almonds. The bold flavors of Romesco pair well with grilled meats, baked fish and roasted vegetables.

Makes: 250 g
Prep time: 10 minutes
Cook time: 15 minutes

- 2 tablespoons extra-virgin olive oil
- 1 large sweet red pepper
- 3 plum tomatoes, cored and cut in half
- 2 garlic cloves
- 35 g pecans
- 1 dried Thai red chili, stem removed
- leaves from a 10-cm rosemary sprig, finely chopped
- 1 tablespoon sherry vinegar
- 2 tablespoons chia seeds, ground in a spice grinder
- 1 teaspoon sea salt

Preheat the oven to 190°C/375°F/Gas 5.

Warm the olive oil in a heavy-based 25-cm frying pan over a medium-high heat until shimmering. Add the red pepper and cook, turning every 2 minutes, until half of its surface is browned. Add the tomato halves skin side down to the pan, along with the garlic. Cook, continuing to turn the pepper, until it is browned on all sides and the garlic begins to color, about 2 minutes. Add the pecans, chili and rosemary, then transfer the pan to the oven and cook until the pepper and tomatoes are quite soft and tender, about 8 minutes. Remove the pan from the oven and allow the contents to cool completely.

Remove and discard the stem and seeds from the red pepper and add the flesh to a blender along with the tomato mixture. Scrape any juices and browned bits from the pan into the blender and add the vinegar, chia seeds, and salt. Blend on a high speed until the mixture is as smooth as it can be, about 45 seconds.

Use the sauce right away, or refrigerate in an airtight container for up to 4 days.

Nutritional analysis per serving (60 g): Calories: 178, Fat: 14 g, Saturated Fat: 2 g, Cholesterol: 0 mg, Fiber: 4 g, Protein: 2 g, Carbohydrates: 10 g, Sodium: 636 mg

Chimichurri

Argentina is known for its high-quality beef, and chimichurri is the traditional local accompaniment for grilled steaks. The sauce's fresh, vibrant flavors are perfect with the richness of red meat, but they're great with poultry too.

Makes: 250 g
Prep time: 10 minutes

- 1 bunch flat-leaf parsley, stems removed
- 2 tablespoons fresh oregano leaves
- 6 garlic cloves
- 4 tablespoons extra-virgin olive oil
- 4 tablespoons apple cider vinegar
- 1 teaspoon ground cumin
- 1 teaspoon sea salt
- ½ teaspoon freshly ground black pepper

Combine all the ingredients in a food processor and pulse until just slightly chunky, about 8 pulses.

Use the chimichurri right away or refrigerate in an airtight container for up to 2 weeks.

Nutritional analysis per serving (60 g): *Calories: 372, Fat: 41 g, Saturated Fat: 6 g, Cholesterol: 0 mg, Fiber: 1 g, Protein: 1 g, Carbohydrates: 2 g, Sodium: 604 mg*

ROSEMARY VINAIGRETTE

Rosemary is a hardy Mediterranean herb that is said to improve memory and is known for its antibacterial properties. Use this robust vinaigrette on salads or fish, or as a marinade for tempeh or chicken.

Makes: about 500 ml
Prep time: 10 minutes

- 375 ml extra-virgin olive oil
- 190 ml apple cider vinegar
- 1 tablespoon wholegrain mustard
- leaves from 1 large sprig fresh rosemary, finely chopped
- 1 garlic clove
- 1 teaspoon sea salt
- ¼ teaspoon freshly ground black pepper

Combine all the ingredients in a blender and blend on high speed until well combined, about 45 seconds.

Use right away or refrigerate in an airtight container for up to 2 weeks. (If refrigerated, bring to room temperature and whisk to recombine before using.)

Nutritional analysis per serving (60 ml): *Calories: 364, Fat: 44 g, Saturated Fat: 8 g, Cholesterol: 0 mg, Fiber: 0 g, Protein: 0 g, Carbohydrates: 0 g, Sodium: 288 mg*

Pine Nut Caesar Dressing

Sometimes I miss a good Caesar dressing for romaine lettuce and other greens. This cheese-free version, which uses pine nuts and nutritional yeast, will fool anyone with its creamy goodness. It is absolutely possible to achieve a rich, supple texture without using dairy.

Makes: about 250 ml
Prep time: 5 minutes

- 75 g pine nuts
- 2 garlic cloves
- 2 tablespoons nutritional yeast
- 1 tablespoon Dijon mustard
- 4 olive oil-packed anchovies
- 2 tablespoons fresh lemon juice
- 4 tablespoons extra-virgin olive oil
- ½ teaspoon sea salt

Combine all the ingredients in a blender and blend on high speed until smooth and creamy, about 1 minute.

Use the dressing right away or refrigerate in an airtight container for up to 1 week.

Nutritional analysis per serving (60 ml): Calories: 427, Fat: 41 g, Saturated Fat: 5 g, Cholesterol: 3 mg, Fiber: 3 g, Protein: 9 g, Carbohydrates: 7 g, Sodium: 522 mg

SOUTHEAST-ASIAN-STYLE ALMOND BUTTER SAUCE

Use this flavorful, easy-to-make sauce with homemade chicken nuggets, or with kelp or courgette noodles, or as a dip for vegetable crudités.

Makes: about 500 ml
Prep time: 5 minutes

- 4 tablespoons full-fat coconut milk
- 190 g roasted almond butter
- 2.5-cm piece fresh ginger, peeled and grated
- 1 garlic clove
- 2 tablespoons wheat-free tamari
- 2 tablespoons fresh lime juice
- 2 tablespoons rice vinegar
- 1 tablespoon fish sauce
- 1 small dried red chili

Combine all the ingredients in a blender and blend on high speed until creamy, about 45 seconds.

Use the sauce right away or transfer to an airtight container and refrigerate for up to 1 week.

Nutritional analysis per serving (2 tablespoons): *Calories: 52, Fat: 3 g, Saturated Fat: 0 g, Cholesterol: 0 mg, Fiber: 1 g, Protein: 2 g, Carbohydrates: 2 g, Sodium: 159 mg*

SMOKY KETCHUP

PEGAN DIET

People always tell me they miss ketchup for spreading on a burger or for dipping chips, so I had to include a Pegan version in this collection of recipes. It's sugar-free and gets a spicy, lightly smoky flavor from chipotle powder.

Makes: 125 ml
Prep time: 5 minutes
Cook time: 20 minutes

- 65 g tomato purée
- 1 small shallot, thinly sliced
- 2 tablespoons apple cider vinegar
- 2 teaspoons Dijon mustard
- ½ teaspoon chipotle powder
- ½ teaspoon ground allspice
- general pinch of ground cloves
- ½ teaspoon sea salt
- 2 dates, pitted

Place all the ingredients in a small, heavy-based saucepan and pour in 375 ml filtered water. Bring to a simmer over a medium heat and cook, stirring occasionally, until the water evaporates and the mixture thickens, 15 to 20 minutes.

Using a stick blender, purée the mixture in the saucepan until smooth. Alternatively, transfer the mixture to a blender and blend on high speed until smooth.

Use the ketchup right away or refrigerate in an airtight container for up to 1 week.

Nutritional analysis per serving (2 tablespoons): *Calories: 60, Fat: 0 g, Saturated Fat: 0 g, Cholesterol: 0 mg, Fiber: 4 g, Protein: 0 g, Carbohydrates: 16 g, Sodium: 652 mg*

GINGERY BARBECUE SAUCE

I love good barbecue sauce, so here's one that has all the right tangy, sweet and spicy flavors, but without any added sugar. It pairs well with chicken, but I also enjoy it slathered on roasted cauliflower, grilled portobello mushrooms, tempeh and tofu.

Makes: 500 ml
Prep time: 15 minutes
Cook time: 1 hour, plus cooling time

- 2 x 400-g cans whole peeled tomatoes
- 2 tablespoons extra-virgin olive oil
- 1 large onion, finely chopped
- 2.5-cm piece fresh ginger, peeled and finely chopped
- 3 garlic cloves, crushed
- 125 ml apple cider vinegar
- 125 ml wheat-free tamari
- 1 whole star anise
- 1 teaspoon ground allspice
- ¼ teaspoon sea salt
- ¼ teaspoon freshly ground black pepper

Purée the tomatoes and their juice. Warm the olive oil in a medium heavy-based saucepan over a medium heat until shimmering. Add the onion and cook, stirring occasionally, until softened and translucent, 4 to 5 minutes. Stir in the ginger and garlic and cook until fragrant, about 2 minutes. Pour in the vinegar and allow to reduce by half. Add 375 ml filtered water and the tamari, star anise, allspice, salt and pepper and simmer, stirring occasionally, until the sauce has thickened and reduced to about 500 ml, about 45 minutes. Allow to cool completely.

Use the sauce right away or refrigerate in an airtight container for up to 5 days.

Nutritional analysis per serving (125 ml): *Calories: 245, Fat: 10 g, Saturated Fat: 0 g, Cholesterol: 0 mg, Fiber: 10 g, Protein: 5 g, Carbohydrates: 45 g, Sodium: 2195 mg*

Classic Tomato Sauce

Every home cook needs a good recipe for tomato sauce. Once you see how simple it is to make and how great the results taste, you'll never buy ready-made sauce again. I like to make large batches and freeze the sauce by the litre.

Makes: 2 litres
Prep time: 5 minutes
Cook time: 8 hours, 20 minutes (mostly unattended)

- 4 x 400-g cans whole peeled tomatoes
- 2 tablespoons extra-virgin olive oil
- 5 garlic cloves, crushed
- 3 tablespoons tomato purée
- 2 teaspoons dried thyme
- 1 teaspoon dried oregano
- 1 bay leaf
- 50 g basil leaves, torn into small pieces
- 2 teaspoons sea salt
- ½ teaspoon freshly ground black pepper

Purée the tomatoes and their juice in a blender until smooth.

Warm the olive oil in a large, heavy-based saucepan over a medium-high heat until shimmering. Add the garlic and cook, stirring frequently, until golden brown, 2 to 3 minutes. Stir in the tomato purée and cook until slightly darkened in color, about 2 minutes. Carefully pour in the puréed tomatoes, add the thyme, oregano and bay leaf, and pour in 2 litres filtered water. Bring to the boil, then cover partially and simmer, stirring occasionally, until the sauce is quite thick, about 8 hours.

Add the basil and continue to simmer to allow the flavors to mingle, about 15 minutes. Stir in the salt and pepper. Use the sauce right away, or store it in an airtight container in the refrigerator for up to 4 days, or freeze for up to 6 months.

Nutritional analysis per serving (125 ml): *Calories: 148, Fat: 8 g, Saturated Fat: 2 g, Cholesterol: 0 mg, Fiber: 8 g, Protein: 4 g, Carbohydrates: 18 g, Sodium: 952 mg*

GHEE

Ghee, the cooking fat of choice in India, has a wonderfully rich flavor and is very simple to make at home using unsalted, grass-fed butter. Unlike ordinary clarified butter, ghee is pure butterfat and free of milk solids, so those with lactose sensitivities usually do fine with ghee. If you'll be using a lot of ghee in your cooking, you can double the recipe and make a bigger batch—ghee keeps for up to 6 months in the refrigerator.

Makes: 450 g
Prep time: 2 minutes
Cook time: 15 minutes

- 450 g unsalted, grass-fed butter, cut into cubes

Warm the butter in a small saucepan over a medium heat until completely melted and beginning to simmer. Reduce the heat to low and cook without stirring until the butter foams and the foam settles at the bottom of the pan, about 15 minutes. Allow to cool slightly.

Line a fine-mesh sieve with several layers of muslin and set the sieve over a bowl. Strain the ghee into the bowl, then transfer to a glass jar and seal tightly.

Store the ghee at room temperature for up to 30 days, or in the refrigerator for up to 6 months.

Nutritional analysis per serving (2 tablespoons): *Calories: 200, Fat: 20 g, Saturated Fat: 14 g, Cholesterol: 60 mg, Fiber: 0 g, Protein: 0 g, Carbohydrates: 0 g, Sodium: 0 mg*

HERBED COMPOUND BUTTER

Compound butter is a fantastic delivery system for rich flavor and good-quality fat. Use this version on Spiced Sweet Potato Quick Bread (page 251), or melt it into Pegan Diet-approved cooked vegetables and grains. Slice 5-mm pats of the chilled butter and place them on fish or chicken before baking, or set them on top of just-cooked steaks and allow to melt over the meat.

Makes: 450 g
Prep time: 15 minutes

- 450 g unsalted, grass-fed butter, cut into cubes, room temperature
- 30 g fresh parsley leaves
- 2 tablespoons fresh mint leaves, roughly chopped
- 1 tablespoon fresh rosemary leaves, finely chopped
- leaves from 2 thyme sprigs, roughly chopped
- 2 teaspoons sea salt
- ¼ teaspoon freshly ground black pepper

Pulse the butter cubes in a food processor to break them up, 4 or 5 pulses. Scrape down the bowl and process until the butter is creamy and smooth, about 45 seconds. Add the herbs, salt and pepper and process until well combined, about 1 minute.

Cut a 30-cm square of baking parchment and lay it on a work surface. Scoop the butter onto the bottom quarter of the parchment and form it into a log about 10 cm long, using the parchment to help you create a compact shape. Wrap the log in the parchment and twist the ends so that the parcel resembles a wrapped toffee. Refrigerate until the butter is firm, at least 2 hours or up to 6 days, or freeze for up to 3 months.

Nutritional analysis per serving (2 tablespoons): *Calories: 212, Fat: 24 g, Saturated Fat: 16 g, Cholesterol: 60 mg, Fiber: 0 g, Protein: 0 g, Carbohydrates: 2 g, Sodium: 290 mg*

Meyer Lemon-Chive Compound Butter

The Meyer lemon, a cross between the common orange and the lemon, has a lemon-like flavor, but with less acidity and a touch more sweetness. Use this compound butter on chicken, fresh wild salmon or halibut. You won't be able to get enough of it!

Makes: 450 g
Prep time: 15 minutes

- 2 garlic cloves
- 1 teaspoon sea salt
- 450 g unsalted, grass-fed butter, cut into small cubes, at room temperature
- grated zest of 4 Meyer lemons
- 2 tablespoons finely chopped fresh chives

Finely chop the garlic, sprinkle it with the salt, and continue to chop until the garlic forms a paste.

Place the butter in a mixer fitted with a flex-edge beater attachment and beat until smooth and creamy, 2 to 3 minutes. Alternatively, whiz the butter in a food processor for 1 minute, then scrape down the sides of the bowl. Add the garlic paste, lemon zest and chives and mix until well combined.

Cut a 30-cm sheet of baking parchment and lay it on a work surface. Scoop the butter onto the bottom quarter of the parchment and form it into a log about 13 cm long, using the parchment to help you create a compact shape. Wrap the log in the parchment and twist the ends so that the parcel resembles a wrapped toffee. Refrigerate until the butter is firm, at least 2 hours or up to 6 days, or freeze for up to 3 months.

Nutritional analysis per serving (2 tablespoons): *Calories: 200, Fat: 22 g, Saturated Fat: 14 g, Cholesterol: 60 mg, Fiber: 0 g, Protein: 0 g, Carbohydrates: 0 g, Sodium: 144 mg*

Pickled Kohlrabi

From sauerkraut to kimchi, naturally pickled, or fermented, vegetables are enjoyed by many cultures around the world. The simple fermentation process below uses kohlrabi, a vegetable in the same family as cabbage and broccoli. The crunchy result goes well with just about any meal.

Makes: 575 g
Prep time: 20 minutes, plus 3 to 4 days for fermentation

- 900 g green or purple kohlrabi
- 2 tablespoons sea salt
- 1 teaspoon ground turmeric

Cut off the top and bottom of the kohlrabi, then peel and quarter the bulbs. In a food processor fitted with the medium shredding disk, shred the kohlrabi. Pack the shreds into a 1-litre, wide-necked jar.

Put 1 litre lukewarm filtered water in a medium bowl or a large measuring jug, add the salt and stir until it has completely dissolved. Stir in the turmeric, then pour the mixture over the kohlrabi, filling the jar to just below the rim.

Cover the jar with a piece of muslin and secure with a rubber band. Leave to stand at room temperature until the liquid becomes bubbly when the jar is gently agitated, 3 to 4 days.

Serve right away or remove the muslin, cover the jar with its lid, and refrigerate for up to 1 month.

Nutritional analysis per serving (140 g): *Calories: 108, Fat: 5 g, Saturated Fat: 2 g, Cholesterol: 0 mg, Fiber: 3 g, Protein: 4 g, Carbohydrates: 11 g, Sodium: 3973 mg*

Fragrant Spice Blend

Having an assortment of spice blends at the ready will allow you to season different cuts of meat with big, bold flavors even when you're pressed for time. This particular blend is perfect for lamb, yet mild enough for use on chicken. To remove the cardamom seeds from the pod, gently crush it against a work surface, then use your fingers to crack it open and remove the seeds.

Makes: 125 g
Prep time: 5 minutes
Cook time: 5 minutes

- 2 tablespoons coriander seeds
- 4 teaspoons cumin seeds
- 2 teaspoons fennel seeds
- 2 small dried red chilies
- seeds from 1 cardamom pod
- 2 tablespoons sea salt

Place the coriander seeds in a small frying pan with the cumin seeds, fennel seeds, chilies and cardamom seeds. Set the pan over a medium–high heat and toast the spices, shaking the pan continuously, until very fragrant, 3 to 4 minutes.

Transfer the spices to a spice grinder and whiz until finely ground and powdery. (Alternatively, use a mortar and pestle to grind the spices.) Transfer the spice mixture to an airtight container and stir in the salt. Use the spice blend right away, or seal the container and store at room temperature for up to 6 months.

Nutritional analysis per serving (2 tablespoons): *Calories: 17, Fat: 1 g, Saturated Fat: 0 g, Cholesterol: 0 mg, Fiber: 2 g, Protein: 0 g, Carbohydrates: 3 g, Sodium: 1683 mg*

Sofrito

Sofrito is the traditional flavor base for many Latin American and Spanish dishes. While sofrito ingredients may differ from region to region, the mixture always contains aromatic vegetables, such as onions, peppers and garlic, which are cooked slowly to concentrate the flavors and allow them to meld. Use sofrito as a seasoning for meats and roasted veggies, or stir some into cooked grains such as rice and quinoa during the Pegan portion of the plan.

Makes: about 1 kg
Prep time: 10 minutes
Cook time: 35 minutes, plus cooling time

- 900 g plum tomatoes, cored and roughly chopped
- 2 large sweet red peppers, seeded and roughly chopped
- 2 large onions, roughly chopped
- 4 large garlic cloves
- 2 tablespoons paprika
- 1 teaspoon smoked paprika
- 2 tablespoons extra-virgin olive oil or rendered lard

Put the tomatoes, peppers, onions and garlic in a large bowl and toss together.

Working in two or three batches, pulse the vegetables in a food processor until finely chopped, 4 or 5 pulses. Transfer to a medium bowl and stir in both types of paprika.

Warm the olive oil in a large saucepan over a medium–high heat until shimmering. Add the vegetable mixture and cook, stirring occasionally, until thickened and reduced to about 1 kg, 25 to 30 minutes.

Allow the sofrito to cool completely. Transfer to an airtight container and refrigerate for up to 2 weeks or freeze for up to 6 months.

Nutritional analysis per serving (125 g): *Calories: 85, Fat: 4 g, Saturated Fat: 1 g, Cholesterol: 0 mg, Fiber: 3 g, Protein: 2 g, Carbohydrates: 14 g, Sodium: 14 mg*

16

7-Day *Eat Fat, Get Thin* Meal Plan

I can talk about the importance of cutting out processed sugars and carbohydrates and eating plenty of plant foods and healthy fats, but everyone wants to know: Do I walk the talk? The truth is, I have to. I have about ten jobs, two kids, a dog, a work team, weeks and weeks of travel at a time, and the list goes on and on. In order to keep up with this lifestyle, maintaining excellent health becomes a top priority. Thankfully, I prefer the taste of real food over processed junk, and once you reap the benefits of optimal health, turning back isn't even an option.

My day usually starts with some movement—a bike ride, a run, a yoga class, or a game of basketball with my son. When I have a long day ahead of me or I am planning on being extra active, I like to have a little Bulletproof Coffee (page 67), which keeps me satiated for hours. I will also have a smoothie or make some eggs or another delicious, full-fat breakfast dish. For lunch, I enjoy salad on weekdays, and on the weekends, if I have time, I'll prepare something a little more intricate. For dinner, we go all out. I love to cook with my son and daughter if they are in town. We invite a group of friends over and enjoy great conversation and amazing food.

I've created a 7-Day Meal Plan to show you what a week on the *Eat Fat, Get Thin* diet looks like. This plan does not need to be followed to the letter. You can make extras of one recipe for leftovers, or you can replace recipes with any other meal that fits your fancy in this book. Overleaf is an example of a meal plan that I might put together when I am at home in Massachusetts. For dinner, I always recommend making multiple side dishes, which you can find starting on page 148. Variety is key for me, so this meal plan has a little bit of everything.

	Monday	Tuesday	Wednesday	Thursday	Friday	Saturday	Sunday
Breakfast	Chocolate-Raspberry Smoothie (page 66)	Buttery Broccoli and Spinach with Fried Eggs (page 71)	Minted Green Smoothie with Raspberries (page 63)	Southwestern Tofu Scramble (page 81)	Creamy Strawberry and Greens Smoothie (page 61)	Walnut Pancakes with Blueberries (page 82)	Mushroom and Egg Scramble (page 77)
Lunch	Chicken and Rocket Salad with Roasted Red Pepper Vinaigrette (page 121)	Taco Salad (page 125)	Mediterranean Sardine Salad (page 120)	Za'atar-Roasted Chicken (page 216)	Hearty Spinach Salad (page 113) + Rich Onion Soup (page 139)	Turkey Burgers with Peppers and Onions (page 220)	Farmers' Market Salad with Miso Dressing (page 108)
Dinner	"Spaghetti" and Meatballs with Tomato Sauce (page 226)	Seared Scallops with Curried Brussels Sprout Slaw (page 193)	Balsamic Beef Stew (page 235) and Shaved Asparagus and Radicchio Salad (page 111)	Thai Red Curry with Seafood and Vegetables (page 196)	Braised Lamb Shanks with Moroccan Flavors (page 248)	Prawns with Sweet Potatoes, Kale, and Coconut Milk (page 191)	Pot Roast (page 233)

SHOPPING LIST FOR THE 7-DAY MEAL PLAN

Fruit

8 ripe Hass avocados
150 g fresh blueberries
3 lemons

3 limes
2 navel oranges

Vegetables

1 bunch asparagus
2 heads broccoli
450 g Brussels sprouts
1 red cabbage
1.75 kg carrots
1 bunch celery

150 g cherry tomatoes
900 g cremini mushrooms
1 large cucumber
2 × 2.5 cm pieces ginger
450 g green beans
1 large sweet green pepper

4 large sweet red peppers
1 bunch radishes
1 large spaghetti squash
2 large summer squash
2 large sweet potatoes
2 large tomatoes
450 g turnips

1 large courgette
5 heads garlic
2 small red onions
1 large shallot
15 large onions
2 bunches spring onions

Greens, Herbs

375 g rocket
900g mixed baby greens
1 bunch cavolo nero
750 g baby spinach
1 head radicchio

1 small bunch fresh rosemary
3 bunches fresh coriander
1 bunch fresh basil
1 bunch fresh thyme
2 bunches flat-leaf parsley

Meat, Fish, Poultry

3 dozen eggs
900 g grass-fed ground beef
750 g beef stew meat
1 × 900-g beef rump roasting
    joint
3.5 kg soup bones
1.5–1.75 kg boneless chicken
    breasts

4 chicken legs
4 lamb shanks
450 g mussels
4 × 120-g cans sardines in
    water or olive oil
750 g scallops
750 g large prawns
450 g turkey

Nuts, Seeds

150 g almonds (for nut milk)
20 g chia seeds
135 g cup hazelnuts
40 g cup hemp seeds

35 g pine nuts
10 g pumpkin seeds
35 g raw sunflower seeds
100 g walnuts

Grocery

2 × 400-ml cans full-fat
    unsweetened coconut milk

500 ml beef stock
1 jar ghee

1 package kombu
1 jar roasted red peppers
1 jar olive oil-marinated
    sun-dried tomatoes
2 × 400-g cans tomatoes
1 × 200-g glass jar tomato pureé
1 × 500 ml bottle tomato passata
1 small jar Dijon mustard
1 small jar whole-grain mustard
400 g pitted Kalamata olives
1 jar red curry paste
1 box peppermint tea bags
1 small bottle red wine vinegar
1 small bottle apple cider
    vinegar

1 jar wheat-free tamari
1 litre extra-virgin olive oil
1 jar coconut oil
1 litre avocado oil
1 small bottle sherry vinegar
1 small bottle balsamic vinegar
1 small bottle fish sauce
1 small bottle liquid smoke
1 small bottle white wine
    vinegar or champagne
    vinegar
450 g coconut flour
225 g arrowroot powder
225 g ounces cacao powder

Spices

450 g sea salt
1 small jar ground white pepper
1 small jar curry powder
1 jar whole black peppercorns
1 small jar cayenne pepper
50 g chipotle powder
50 g chili powder
50 g ground cinnamon
50 g ground coriander seed
50 g ground cumin
1 small jar fennel seeds
1 small jar garlic powder
1 small jar red chili flakes
1 small container saffron threads
1 small jar turmeric

1 small jar dried thyme
1 small jar dried oregano
1 small jar za'atar seasoning
1 jar bay leaves
1 teaspoon vanilla powder
1 small bottle alcohol- and,
    gluten-free pure vanilla
    flavoring
1 small container aluminium-
    free baking powder
1 small container baking soda

Refrigerated Items

450 g unsalted, grass-fed butter
1 block firm (organic, non-
   GMO) tofu

1 jar soy-free miso
   (Clearspring)

Specialty

1 preserved lemon
1 bottle MCT oil (page 27)

1 bottle organic dry white wine
1 bottle organic red wine

Frozen

ice cubes
1 × 350-g pack frozen raspberries
1 × 350-g pack frozen strawberries

Acknowledgments

My vision for this cookbook was to prove once and for all that food can taste good and be good for you *and* that we can and should have healthy relationships with our bodies, our kitchens, and the food we eat. Even though the misguided advice to avoid fats and embrace processed carbohydrates we've heard for decades is still being preached by many doctors, scientists, and even the media, the response to *Eat Fat, Get Thin* has proved to me that we are no longer interested in tasteless, low-fat meals and outdated research. Achieving real, lasting results with real food and enjoying the process is what this book is all about.

This vision would not be possible without you — without anyone who believes that they can transform their health with the power of food. In order to change the health of the world, we need to start with ourselves, so thank *you* for investing in this journey with me.

To help create these deeply satisfying and delectable meals, I knew that I had to find a chef who shared my affection for healthy fats and real, whole foods. My friend Chef Frank Giglio is the first person I thought of. I have never tasted a recipe of his that I didn't love. He has spent a great deal of time creating mouthwatering meals that are designed for maximum nutrition.

For bringing these recipes to life, I'd like to thank our photographer, Leela Cyd, and food stylist Ayda Robana, as well as their teams for capturing all of these beautiful meals. I want to give special thanks to Kaya Purohit, who worked tirelessly on every page, making this book great. I could not do half of what I do without you. Thank you. And, of course,

Dhru Purohit, my business partner, who steers the ship, leads the troops, and makes it all happen!

Of course, none of this would be possible without the people who have kept this book organized—my team at Little, Brown, especially my editor, Tracy Behar, and Jean Garnett. I'd also like to thank my agent, Richard Pine, as well as the Hyman Digital team and my team at The UltraWellness Center and the Cleveland Clinic Center for Functional Medicine for their tremendous amount of support and for helping me spread the message that food *is* medicine.

Resources

FURTHER READING AND RESOURCES FROM MARK HYMAN, MD

Mark Hyman's Websites
www.drhyman.com
www.eatfatgetthin.com
www.10daydetox.com
www.bloodsugarsolution.com

Books and Programs
Eat Fat, Get Thin (book and public television special)
The Blood Sugar Solution 10-Day Detox Diet (book and public television special)
The Blood Sugar Solution 10-Day Detox Diet Cookbook (book)
The Blood Sugar Solution (book and public television special)
The Blood Sugar Solution Cookbook (book)
The UltraMind Solution (book and public television special)
Six Weeks to an UltraMind (audio/DVD program)
The Daniel Plan (book)
The Daniel Plan Cookbook (book)
UltraCalm (audio program)
UltraMetabolism (book and public television special)
The UltraMetabolism Cookbook (book)
The UltraSimple Diet (book)

The UltraThyroid Solution (e-book)
UltraPrevention (book)
The Five Forces of Wellness (audio program)
The Detox Box (audio/DVD program)
Nutrigenomics (audio program)

General References and Resources

Eat Fat, Get Thin Resources

For quizzes, supplement protocol, tracking tools, and all other recommendations, head to www.eatfatgetthin.com/resources, where you will find everything you need.

Pesticide Action Network UK

www.pan-uk.org

A charity that promotes safe and sustainable alternatives to hazardous pesticides. Its website includes a list of the best and worst foods in forms of food residues. It also monitors what actions supermarkets are taking to address pesticide and residue issues.

Index

Recipe Index

About the Author

Mark Hyman, MD, believes that we all deserve a life of vitality—and that we have the potential to create it for ourselves. That's why he is dedicated to tackling the root causes of chronic disease by harnessing the power of Functional Medicine to transform health care. Dr. Hyman and his team work every day to empower people, organizations, and communities to heal their bodies and minds and to improve our social and economic resilience.

Dr. Hyman is a practicing family physician, a ten-time *New York Times* bestselling author, and an internationally recognized leader, speaker, educator, and advocate in his field. He is the Pritzker Foundation Chair in Functional Medicine at Cleveland Clinic and the director of the Cleveland Clinic Center for Functional Medicine. He is also the founder and director of The UltraWellness Center, chairman of the board of the Institute for Functional Medicine, a medical editor of *The Huffington Post,* and he has been a regular medical contributor on many television shows and networks, including *CBS This Morning, Today, Good Morning America,* CNN, *The View, Katie,* and *The Dr. Oz Show.*

Dr. Hyman works with individuals and organizations, as well as policy makers and influencers. He has testified before both the White House Commission on Complementary and Alternative Medicine and the Senate Working Group on Health Care Reform on Functional Medicine. He has consulted with the surgeon general on diabetes prevention, and participated in the 2009 White House Forum on Prevention and Wellness. Senator Tom Harkin of Iowa nominated Dr. Hyman for the President's

Advisory Group on Prevention, Health Promotion, and Integrative and Public Health. In addition, Dr. Hyman has worked with President Bill Clinton, presenting at the Clinton Foundation's Health Matters, Achieving Wellness in Every Generation conference, and the Clinton Global Initiative, as well as with the World Economic Forum on global health issues. He is the winner of the Linus Pauling Award and the Nantucket Project Award, was inducted into the Books for a Better Life Hall of Fame, and received the Christian Book of the Year Award for *The Daniel Plan.*

Dr. Hyman also works with fellow leaders in his field to help people and communities thrive—with Rick Warren, Dr. Mehmet Oz, and Dr. Daniel Amen, he created The Daniel Plan, a faith-based initiative that helped the Saddleback Church collectively lose 115,000 kg. He is an advisor and guest cohost on *The Dr. Oz Show* and is on the board of Dr. Oz's HealthCorps, which tackles the obesity epidemic by educating American students about nutrition. With Dr. Dean Ornish and Dr. Michael Roizen, Dr. Hyman crafted and helped introduce the Take Back Your Health Act of 2009 to the United States Senate to provide for reimbursement of lifestyle treatment of chronic disease. And with Tim Ryan in 2015, he helped introduce the ENRICH Act into Congress to fund nutrition in medical education. Dr. Hyman plays a substantial role in a major film produced by Laurie David and Katie Couric, released in 2014, called *Fed Up,* which addresses childhood obesity. Please join him in helping us all to take back our health at drhyman.com, and follow him on Twitter (@markhymanmd), Facebook (facebook.com/drmarkhyman), and Instagram (@markhymanmd).